BACK PAIN

BRIDGING THE GAP
BETWEEN MIND AND BODY

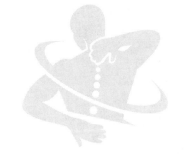

KUSAL
GOONEWARDENA

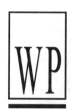

Published by Wilkinson Publishing Pty Ltd
ACN 006 042 173
PO Box 24135, Melbourne, VIC 3001, Australia
Ph: +61 3 9654 5446
enquiries@wilkinsonpublishing.com.au
www.wilkinsonpublishing.com.au

Cover and book design by Jo Hunt
Images sourced from Shutterstock.
Printed and bound in Australia by Ligare Pty Ltd.

ISBN: 9781925927788

A catalogue record for this book is available from the
National Library of Australia.

Follow Wilkinson Publishing on social media.

WilkinsonPublishing
wilkinsonpublishinghouse
WPBooks

CONTENTS

IS YOUR LIFE ON HOLD?

Our enthusiasm for life can come to a painful halt when physical limitations put an offending barrier on our spirit, not allowing us to experience new thrills and adventure. Every person, without fail, wants to share the joys and pleasures in life, with many getting that envied sense of delight and emancipation through experience. And there is nothing more frustrating than when our own body thwarts that ambition.

Lower back pain has engulfed millions in its vicious wrap and continues to do so every day. The good news is that there is a solution. Read on if you have that urge to go out and live your life to the hilt but feel handicapped with lower back pain playing spoilsport! Help is at hand.

While you keep a keen eye on the signs, your body is giving you, forge ahead with the remedies offered in this book. Your lower back pain is not the end of the world because there are methods that lead the way to safe recovery and healing. You will once again relish the true joys of living without physical limitations, putting a dampener on your cherished zest for a great life.

INTRODUCTION

A typical definition of lower back pain (LBP) would be a sudden, sharp, persistent or dull pain felt below the waist. Your back is one of the most sensitive yet heavily used parts of the body, so it is easy to injure, and it carries a considerable burden of responsibility for keeping you living your life to the fullest. With early signs of pain in the lumbar region or the lower back, you begin to see the first signs of the wear and tear that this complicated structure has been going through and the first cry for help.

In fact, lower back pain is one of the very few forms of pain that can hugely vary in its intensity. The pain in your lower back can often range from mild, dull and annoying to disabling pain that is persistent and intense. While the first type might cause you to dismiss the signals as mere discomfort, the latter category of pain can be severely debilitating and strongly interfere with your routine or preferred functioning.

The Time Factor

The most conspicuous and significant fact about lower back pain is that it might not develop suddenly or in a short time or be due to any one prominent reason. Instead, the condition might develop over a long course of time after you've been performing many physical activities in the wrong manner, such as sitting, standing, sleeping, lifting and the like. However, once a triggering incident occurs, such as a sudden fall, jerk, or accident, there is an immediate onset of the pain.

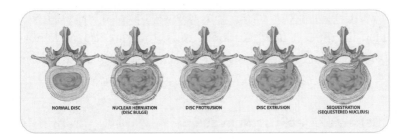

Lower Back—The Structure

The human spine is one of the most complex structures comprising a series of components that each have an essential function. The spine performs the all-important role of giving shape and structure to the body and providing all the necessary support. It is primarily for this reason that an episode of lower back pain can hinder your efficiency in daily life as nothing else can.

When attempting to understand what exactly is happening to your body as you suffer from LBP and why it is happening to you, you must understand the basic structure of the spine.

The human spine has many small bones, known as vertebrae, that stack one on top of the other. The following is a brief introduction of various parts of the human spine.

1. VERTEBRAE

The vertebrae are small bones that interconnect to create a canal that protects the spinal cord. The spinal column comprises three sections that make natural curves in the back. They are:

Neck area (Cervical)
Chest area (Thoracic)
Lower back (Lumbar)

So, the lower section of the spine is where the vertebrae are fused. Here lies the core of a lot of strain issues. There are also five lumbar vertebrae that connect the upper spine to the pelvis at the bottom of the lower back.

2. SPINAL CORD AND NERVES

These are the electrical cables that travel through the spinal canal and carry messages between the brain and muscles. It is through openings in the vertebrae that the nerves flow out from the spinal cord.

3. MUSCLES AND LIGAMENTS

The muscles and ligaments offer support and stability to the spine and the upper body. Strong ligaments perform the critical function of connecting your vertebrae and helping to keep the spinal column in its correct position.

4. FACET JOINTS

In between the vertebrae, small joints help the spine to move. They make the body more flexible and supple. These facet joints are incredibly close to the spinal nerves.

5. INTERVERTEBRAL DISCS

These are the tiny components of the human spine that sit in between the vertebrae. When you run or walk, these intervertebral discs act as shock absorbers and prevent the vertebrae from rubbing against each other. Along with the facet joints, they perform the function of helping the spine to move, twist and bend.

The intervertebral discs have two main components. They have cool Latin names:

Annulus fibrosus, which is the rigid and flexible outer ring of the disc, and Nucleus pulposus, which is the soft, jelly-like centre of the annulus fibrosus, giving the disc its shock-absorbing capabilities.

Back Pain—The Epidemic

If you have suffered from the severe impact of lower back pain then you are not alone—it impacts a significant segment of the world population. The National Institutes of Health (NIH) reports that at least 75–85% of people will suffer from lower back pain at least once in their lifetime. The reports also state that back pain is the most frequent cause of below-normal activity levels in adults younger than 45.

Lower back pain appears to be assuming almost epidemic proportions in the last few years. It matches concerns about increased instances of undesirable lifestyles and overall drooping health standards. In the US alone a whopping 66% of adults suffer from recurring back pain, with numbers looking to be on an upward trend.

Let's keep going with some Canadian statistics. Current research suggests that eight out of every ten Canadians suffer from lower back pain at some point in their life. It is the second leading cause of time loss at work in Canada and costs more from loss of work time than any other reason. Another study reports lower back pain is the cause of expenditure amounting to a staggering $16 billion out of a total of $27 billion incurred on musculoskeletal problems.

PATIENT ACTION CHART

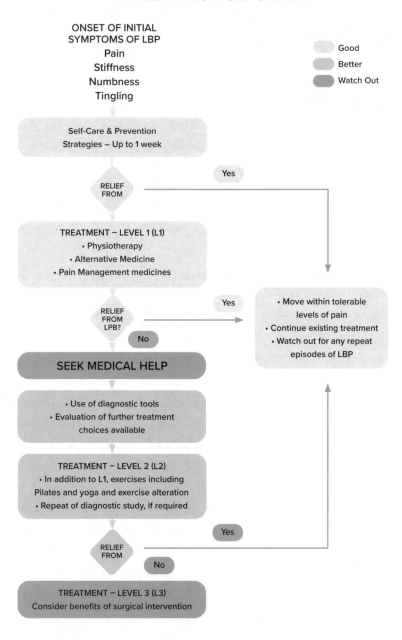

ONSET OF INITIAL
SYMPTOMS OF LBP
Pain
Stiffness
Numbness
Tingling

Good
Better
Watch Out

Self-Care & Prevention
Strategies – Up to 1 week

RELIEF
FROM

Yes

TREATMENT – LEVEL 1 (L1)
• Physiotherapy
• Alternative Medicine
• Pain Management medicines

RELIEF
FROM
LPB?

Yes

No

• Move within tolerable
levels of pain
• Continue existing treatment
• Watch out for any repeat
episodes of LBP

SEEK MEDICAL HELP

• Use of diagnostic tools
• Evaluation of further treatment
choices available

TREATMENT – LEVEL 2 (L2)
• In addition to L1, exercises including
Pilates and yoga and exercise alteration
• Repeat of diagnostic study, if required

RELIEF
FROM

Yes

No

TREATMENT – LEVEL 3 (L3)
Consider benefits of surgical intervention

Your Action Plan

Correct and timely decisions taken now can save you a lot of suffering later and might even help in a speedy recovery from an episode of lower back pain. There needs to be an effective action plan. So, let's chart what to do to deal with pain from when the symptoms first start.

The patient action chart shows how to deal with the issues, but to achieve the desired results, communication between the patient and the physician needs to be effective. The openness and clarity of communication between the two need to be established and maintained as a foundation for a successful treatment plan for lower back pain. There is no escaping the power of working with the support of professionals.

PATIENT CHART		THERAPIST CHART	
Inputs to Doctor	Primary Responsibility	Inputs to Patient	Primary Responsibility
Detail of symptoms, basis Back Pain Journal (ref. Appendix) Detail of medical history	Compliance of physician's instructions Convey honest feedback about treatment Regular visits to convey feedback Regular self-care	To give full knowledge of the working of spine/ lower back Explanation of exact cause To give complete knowledge of the treatment plan	To accept details of feedback and alter treatment plan, if required To give the patient a true picture of the state of health

Self-Analysis

Lower back pain can become a very intimidating condition for someone not too familiar with the anatomy of the human body and the lower back in general. In such situations, you should make a note of the most prominent signs and symptoms. Once you have the record of these symptoms, you can then report them to your healthcare provider, who will then diagnose the type of pain you have along with the corrective measures you need to take.

You can use the Back Pain Journal (see page 151) to record your health patterns and critical signs. Take it to your physician who can then understand and analyse your condition well. In addition, you can use the journal to map the self-analysis of your ailment and chart the improvements as you go along.

CHAPTER 1

LOWER BACK PAIN —TYPES, SIGNS AND SYMPTOMS

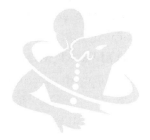

Types of Lower Back Pain

As we now know, lower back pain is one of the most widespread forms of pain-related disorders. It leads to a vast range and variation in the form of pain that occurs. We can understand it by looking at different parameters.

The following section briefly outlines various types of lower back pain based on the pain's duration, cause and location.

A) BASIS OF DURATION

The duration of pain is the most commonly used method to differentiate between different types of lower back pain. In fact, the time scale of the pain and its severity helps the physician decide on the exact cause of the pain and the treatment modalities required.

The following is a description of each of the three types of lower back pain based on their duration.

- **Acute pain** is a short-term pain, mostly lasting from a few days to a few weeks (basically four weeks maximum). Symptoms associated with acute back pain can sometimes become serious if left untreated.
- **Sub-Acute pain** is a moderate level of pain that lasts anywhere between 4–12 weeks and presents itself in occasional flare-ups of pain.
- **Chronic pain** typically lasts for more than three months. This form of pain might be progressive, i.e. it might develop gradually over time. Alternatively, this form of pain might suddenly increase to a higher level after short gaps and then the level of pain might return to normal.

B) BASIS OF TREATMENT MODALITIES

Based on generally required plans, experts suggest two different types of lower back pain. They are mechanical pain and inflammatory pain—both are sub-divisions of non-specific pain, also known as NS-LBP.

Why the pain in my back?—The latest clinical findings

The latest research about understanding pain shows that it is more of a signal by the brain that something is not working correctly in the body. In short, pain in the body works very much like the red engine dashboard light in a car. When the engine is not functioning correctly the light on the dashboard lights up. So when it lights up, we naturally assume something is wrong with the machine. Therefore we take the car to the mechanic and they help fix the engine and stop the red dashboard light.

When you suffer from back pain, it is the same thing—the red engine dashboard light is in the back. To fix the light, we have to fix the engine. The engine is the whole body. In the past, many back pain sufferers naturally thought that their problem is in the lower back. That means that most of the treatment has occurred here. However, in as many as 75% of cases, the problem occurs elsewhere, other than the back. In only 25% of cases the problem that causes the pain occurs in the lower back.

Signs and Symptoms

Lower back pain symptoms are usually directly dependent on ignoring the underlying problem. The worst symptoms occur when ignoring the problem the longest. For example, if the cause of the back pain was a tight joint in the upper spine, and it is ignored, or gets intermittent, short-term treatment, then the signs and symptoms can get much worse.

There are three phases to the signs and symptoms a person may feel. First, they may notice tightness or stiffness in the lower back (people tend to ignore this). Then the body continues to warn the person by only allowing apprehensive movements. For example, a person who wants to bend forward and tie their shoelaces will feel uncomfortable moving down quickly into the position they want. That is apprehension (and is usually also ignored as a symptom). Finally comes the pain, which is when people typically start to think that something is wrong. By this time, however, they are further down the injury path than they know.

The good news is it might not be too late to find a solution.

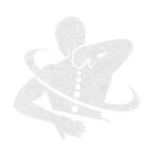

> ### Did you know?
> A frequent observation is that the severity of LBP symptoms might not correlate directly with the severity of the problem. It implies that powerful symptoms might not essentially indicate that any intense underlying disorder exists. For instance, a simple muscle strain might cause extreme pain, while on the other hand, a disc that is wholly degenerated might not cause any pain at all.

Common Symptoms

There are many symptoms of LBP that are pretty general and occur in almost all of the cases. The most prominent amongst these include:

- Severe pain
- Stiffness
- Tingling
- Numbness

Also, pain that:

- Radiates towards buttocks or legs
- Worsens while coughing, twisting, sneezing or after sitting for a prolonged duration.

Specific Symptoms

Lower Back Pain signs and symptoms usually emanate from three primary causes, indicating the exact location of the problem. The following are the actual symptoms of LBP in specific correlation with each of these conditions:

1. SIGNS ASSOCIATED WITH MUSCLE STRAINS AND JOINT STIFFNESS

Being the most common cause of LBP, injuries and sprains in the muscles present the most prominent symptoms. Such an injury or sprain of the muscle usually presents in the form of the following symptoms:

- Muscle spasms
- Stiffness, at times inability to move
- Pain in the gluteal region or buttocks
- Pain that aggravates with specific movements but feels better with rest
- Very tight muscles on either side of the lower spine.

If your LBP emanates from a muscle strain, the pain will typically last from one to three days. This period will then be followed by a few days or weeks of moderate pain as the inflammation diminishes and the affected portion begins to heal.

2. SIGNS ASSOCIATED WITH NERVE ROOT PRESSURE

If your LBP is due to nerve root pressure then the most prominent symptom is that the pain travels down the sciatic nerve in the back of the leg, also known as sciatica or radiculopathy. The most conspicuous signs of the pain caused by nerve root compression include:

- Pain or a heavy feeling in the leg that may also include numbness, tingling, weakness or loss of specific reflexes
- Pain and a heavy sensation that is present only on one side
- Pain that aggravates due to long periods of sitting or standing
- Pain that is quite sharp accompanied by a burning sensation.

The Red Flags

Though lower back pain can rarely be a cause of panic or alarm, there are many red flags or warning signs that need immediate medical attention in case they surface. The most critical warning signs, also known as the 'red flags', include:

- Back pain accompanied by loss of bladder or bowel control
- Loss of sensation in the legs or arms
- Numbness around the genitals, buttocks or anus
- Pain that aggravates when you cough or bend forward from the waist
- Pain that radiates down the leg, towards the knee
- Presence of high fever, which is an indicator of a spinal infection
- Pain that travels up towards the chest
- Severe pain with weight loss, caused by a tumour in the spine
- Severe fever, nausea, vomiting, abdominal pain, weakness or sweating
- Treatment showing negligible effect or no effect after 2–3 weeks.

In addition, individuals who meet the following conditions and suffer from frequent episodes of lower back pain also need to seek medical help immediately. This criterion includes individuals who are:

- Under 20 or over 55 years of age
- Suffered from a recent accident, injury or trauma
- Consumed steroids for a few months
- Drug Abusers
- Those who are suffering or have suffered from cancer
- Those with a low immune system due to treatments like chemotherapy or diseases including HIV/AIDS.

Risk Factors

Research shows that a majority of adults experience lower back pain at some point in their lives. However, a specific group of individuals is more prone to episodes of LBP. Here are the main risk factors which make someone more vulnerable to developing LBP:

- Employees in construction jobs or other places involving heavy lifting
- Employees in any job that involves lots of bending, twisting or vibration of the whole body, such as those using a sandblaster
- People who maintain poor postural habits over a long period. For example, passive postures like working at your computer for 2–6 hours
- Pregnant women
- Individuals over the age of 30, especially those having an unhealthy lifestyle
- Individuals who do not exercise regularly or are overweight
- Individuals who smoke regularly
- People with arthritis or osteoporosis
- People with anxiety or depression
- Individuals with a low pain tolerance level.

CHAPTER 2

KEY CAUSES OF LOWER BACK PAIN

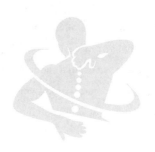

Have you ever suffered intense bouts of lower back pain but have felt helpless when understanding the exact cause? The fact is that in many cases, lower back pain is not a disorder in itself but often a symptom of another disease or malfunction.

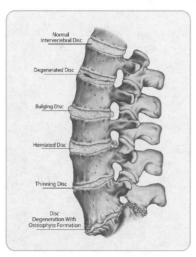

It is essential to know how your body and bones react to the ageing process to understand how lower back pain finds its roots in your body. As your age progresses, there is a significant drop in the levels of bone strength and muscle elasticity. Soon after, the discs start to lose their flexibility and the fluid levels begin to diminish. Eventually this decreases the ability of your discs to cushion the vertebrae appropriately.

Beyond a series of detailed analysis and research findings, sudden, improper use of the postural muscles emerges as the single most common reason for LBP. When you do not engage in the proper posture when performing tasks that require extra effort, the result is a sudden onset of pain in the back. Such activities could span a vast range from playing a random tennis game, gardening, lifting heavy furniture, having a fall or a car accident.

Below are multiple activities, medical conditions and disorders that might cause LBP under different sub-categories to give you a better understanding.

A) INJURIES AND ACTIVITIES

Your back bears the direct impact of your physical activity and will present an immediate effect in case of any injury or accident. In fact, our clinical work reports that at least 75% of cases of lower back pain occur due to neural, muscular or joint tightness in another part of the body. In everyday life, five crucial and common causes mark the onset of lower back pain for most individuals. These include:

- Improper conditioning of the postural muscles
- Improper lifting techniques
- Sprains and injuries of the ligaments and muscles, such as lumbosacral strain, intervertebral joint injuries and rupture of intervertebral discs
- A sudden impact such as from car accidents.

B) NERVE ROOT COMPRESSION

Various medical conditions or disorders in the human body can lead to additional pressure put on the nerve roots in the spinal canal. It can lead to mild or more vigorous episodes of lower back pain, lasting for varying durations.

Your lower back pain could be a result of nerve root compression if you are diagnosed with any of the following medical conditions:

Herniated/Bulging Disc

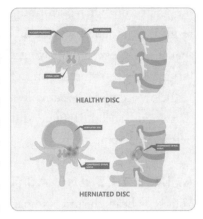

Individuals involved in repetitive activities having a lot of vibration or motion are prone to developing a herniated disc. If you've extensively used machinery or do a specific sports activity requiring heavy physical exertion or have attempted to lift a heavy object using inappropriate lifting techniques, you may be suffering from a herniated disc, which in turn might be an underlying cause of your lower back pain.

Osteoarthritis

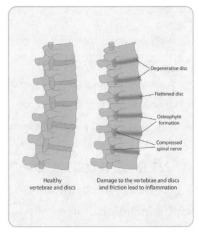

Also known as joint degeneration, osteoarthritis is mainly related to age and affects the small facet joints in the spine, ultimately leading to episodes of lower back pain. Interestingly, research shows that osteoarthritis affects nearly three times as many women as men.

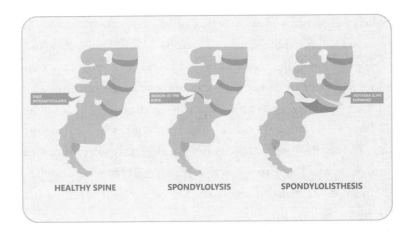

HEALTHY SPINE   SPONDYLOLYSIS   SPONDYLOLISTHESIS

Spondylolysis

This category of physical disorder is a vertebra defect that can allow a vertebra to slide over another one and lead to pain in the back. This particular condition gets aggravated due to specific physical activities that might put stress on the affected regions.

Lumbar Spinal Stenosis

Spinal stenosis is a medical condition that occurs when the space around the spinal cord gets narrowed. It puts further pressure on the spinal cord and the spinal nerve roots, eventually leading to pain, numbness or weakness in the legs.

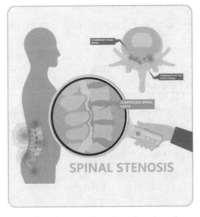

SPINAL STENOSIS

When spinal stenosis occurs in the lower back, the lumbar spinal stenosis usually results from the normal aging process. With age, the soft tissues and bones in the spine harden on their own or become overgrown. Such degenerative changes may narrow the space around the spinal cord and eventually cause spinal stenosis.

In addition, other conditions such as fractures of the vertebrae and spinal deformities such as curvature problems could also cause compression on the nerve roots, further leading to lower back pain.

Nerve root irritation occurs most commonly when a structure next to the nerve becomes dysfunctional (e.g. swollen, inflamed and/or spasmed) due to protective guarding. It often occurs when the nerve roots first exit your spine: at the neck for the arms and the lower back for the legs.

When nerve irritation is not tested and fixed, it can be the most significant reason for the slow recovery from pain and injury—and recurring pain and injury.

How does nerve irritation feel?

Commonly, nerve irritation can cause symptoms such as:

- Radiating pain down the arm or the leg
- Muscle guarding, spasm, or cramping
- Numbness
- Pins and needles
- Aches that do not ease with pain medication
- Difficulty finding a comfortable, pain-free position
- Latent pain/tightness in response to stretching, posture, or activity, and
- No pain, but a tightness that does not loosen up (e.g. in the neck, back, hamstrings).

What is not commonly known is that nerve irritation can be a significant contributing factor to any musculoskeletal or sports pain, stiffness, or injury, with or without the symptoms above. Each person's experience of symptoms will often be different from case to case. Consequences of untreated nerve root irritation include:

- Slower healing and recovery
- Treatments applied do not hold well
- Smaller improvements or none at all
- High chance of injury recurrence.

These are the main reasons why I always look to assess and treat nerve root irritation first.

What can you do to help resolve your nerve irritation?

Nerves are the most sensitive structures in the body; thus, resolving any nerve irritation requires a gentle approach. Unfortunately, conventional exercises that you might use to release a tight muscle or joint (e.g. stretches) are ineffective at treating nerve root irritation. In fact, in most cases, it can lead to the irritation getting worse.

An experienced physiotherapist can help you resolve the nerve irritation anywhere in the body by using specialised hands-on techniques in session. Once you leave the clinic, the best course of action is to prevent re-aggravation of the nerves through activity limitation and having a minimal delay between further sessions. You should only need to limit your regular activities in the early stages of recovery.

In severe cases, prescribed medication may be helpful. If nerve irritation does not resolve quickly with the hands-on techniques, your physiotherapist will help you find alternate solutions to fix it.

For most cases, until you fix the nerve irritation, the following rules apply:

- NO stretching
- NO exercise or limited exercise as guided by your physiotherapist
- DO NOT sit for longer than necessary
- DO NOT use the arm or leg in a stretched-out position. Example: No feet-up while sitting, no striding out with walking, no reaching behind to the back seat, no carrying in that arm or over that shoulder
- DO NOT prop your head up with pillows to read/use a computer while lying on your back (it is better to be lying on your side to read or having the laptop up high enough on cushions, so you don't have to prop up your head)
- For the times you must sit, ensure you use the best possible ergonomic position, sit on a firm chair (like a dining chair) and no sitting on couches
- For the times you must drive, ensure the seat is as close to the pedals as practical. Make sure that your elbows are bent as you drive. Where possible, get someone to drive for you, especially if you are having troubles using the stick or pedals
- When you walk, take small steps, and do your best to avoid limping.

After recovery from your nerve root irritation, your physiotherapist can show you how to prevent recurrence; in most cases, this will require some changes to postural habits or improvement of technique during certain activities.

C) SPINAL CONDITIONS

In addition to the above causes, other medical conditions, specifically related to the spine, result in lower back pain in some individuals. However, the incidence is not very high. Read on for a brief description of each of these conditions:

- Spinal tumours: These are growths that develop on the spine or nerve roots' bones and ligaments
- Metastatic tumours from other points such as prostate, lungs, kidney, and intestine
- Ankylosing spondylitis, which is a kind of arthritis that mainly affects the spine
- Bacterial infections, such as osteomyelitis, which is an infection of the bone or other diseases in the spinal discs or spinal cord occurring due to IV drug use, surgeries or other injection treatments
- Paget's disease, leading to abnormal bone growth, which further affects the pelvis, spine, skull, cheat and lungs
- Scheuermann's disease: A disorder in which one or more vertebrae begin to develop wedge-shaped deformities, leading to further conditions like curvature in the spine, eventually leading to lower back pain.

D) FUNCTIONAL PROBLEMS

Lower back pain can often occur due to several functional issues associated with everyday life activities. Here I've listed some of the most common practical problems causing lower back pain:

- Pregnancy, childbirth, and gynecological operations
- Uterus prolapse
- Pelvic inflammatory diseases
- Cancerous lesions in the pelvic regions
- Endometriosis
- Obesity
- Short leg (on one side)

E) OTHER CONDITIONS

Some of the other conditions that might cause lower back pain include:

- Peptic ulcers
- Aortic aneurysm
- Gallbladder disease
- Pancreatitis
- Cauda equine syndrome
- Urinary disorders
- Kidney disorders
- Biliary stones
- Prostate disease

Causes of Lower Back Pain

Injuries and Activities

1. Improper conditioning of postural muscles

2. Improper lifting techniques

3. Sprains and injuries of ligaments and muscles

4. Sudden impact

Nerve Root Compression

1. Herniated disc

2. Osteoarthritis

3. Spondylolysis

4. Lumbar Spinal Stenosis

5. Sciatica

Spinal Conditions

1. Spinal and metastatic tumours

2. Ankylosing Spondylities

3. Bacterial infections, e.g. Osteomyelitis

4. Paget's disease

5. Scheuermann's disease

Others

1. Peptic ulcers

2. Aortic aneurysm

3. Gallbladder disease

4. Pancreatitis

5. Cauda equine syndrome

6. Urinary disorders

7. Kidney disorders

8. Biliary stones

9. Prostate disease

CHAPTER 3

SELF-CARE AND PREVENTION

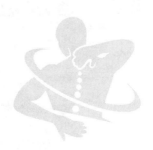

A) SELF-CARE

Medical research consistently reinforces the need for better preventive measures rather than rigorous treatment methods. Even in your everyday life, you should follow precautions and preventative measures to avoid causing a strain on your back.

Read on for some of the essential points to remember to avoid hurting your back and suffering bouts of lower back pain.

Preventive Measures

- Remember not to bend while trying to lift something from the ground. Instead, try to bend your knees and squat to pick up an object. Keeping your back straight, hold the thing you are picking up close to your body and then try to lift it
- While moving heavy objects, try to push instead of pull

- Take frequent breaks to stretch if you need to sit at your desk or drive for longer durations of time
- Follow a regular regimen for exercise as a sedentary and inactive lifestyle contributes to lower back pain substantively.

Curative Measures

- Remain as active as possible during LBP. Prolonged periods of bed rest are known to be a causative factor of lower back pain
- Follow a home exercise program soon after the initial pain has subsided
- Use a heat pad or ice pack (whichever helps you the most) to relieve your pain, especially in the first few weeks
- Lumbar supports such as back support, corsets, and braces might also help alleviate pain
- Try to sleep with a pillow placed between or under your knees
- During an attack of acute back pain, try to practice deep breathing. Rhythmic and slow breathing calms the mind, allowing the body to enter into a more relaxed state
- Try to perform light stretching exercises several times a day.

Experts strongly warn about creating an unduly stressful environment for your lower back pain. Worrying in excess over how bad your pain is when it will heal and how much it will affect your efficiency will harm you all the more instead of offering any healing benefits.

Experts strongly warn about creating an unduly stressful environment for your lower back pain. Worrying in excess over how bad your pain is when it will heal and how much it will affect your efficiency will harm you all the more instead of offering any healing benefits.

B) POSTURE MANAGEMENT

As you rush around the day performing the essential duties of your working or life tasks, there are several postures you take, which, if faulty, can lead to lower back pain. The most common postures that need attention include sitting, standing, sleeping and walking.

Sitting and Standing

We estimate that around 90% of back pain injuries we treat in the clinic relate to one key issue that many of us either forget, become used to, or overlook—incorrect posture. For many, posture is a hidden health and fitness issue because people are often unaware that they have posture problems in the first place.

The fit and healthy are not immune. In fact, good posture might be the difference between good and elite performance—your posture has to perform when the body is under load, through training, competing and opposition pressure.

What is good posture? Imagine a piece of string pulling you up from your head. We naturally elongate. You are NOT standing to attention. You are simply standing tall with your shoulders relaxed back, not pulled back.

People tend to stand in two ways: first is with the bum 'sticking' out'—many dancers do this because their pelvis is tilted forwards through habit; the second standing with the bum 'tucked'. In the second scenario, the pelvis tilts backwards.

Imagine your pelvis as a fruit bowl that needs to stay level. Do not let your fruit bowl tip forward (anatomical term—anterior pelvic tilt) or tip backward (anatomically—posterior pelvic tilt). When it's level, it is neutral.

But there is more to posture than standing, and we are seeing more problems with sitting posture as many of us live more sedentary lifestyles. Let's have a look at the six key things anyone can do to improve their sitting and standing posture:

1. Repetition

It takes approximately 3,000 reps of straightening your spine (standing/sitting tall) for this to become automated by the brain. It is what we classify as motor learning. When motor learning occurs, a task becomes automated. For example, golfers try to automate their movements through practice—being a technical sport it takes about 10,000 reps (swings) to automate a golf swing. Standing tall and straightening your spine is not technical, thus it only requires 3,000 reps.

Using the 3,000 reps rule means if you do 200 reps per day, you will achieve good posture in as little as 15 days. So how do you achieve 200 reps per day?

2. Team up

As with exercise, excellent results occur by having allies on board. You may have a partner, family member, child, friend, or colleague who also wants to work on their posture. Together, you can support and remind each other to stand or sit tall: every time you remind someone, you remember too.

> ## Cues to remind you to 'grow tall'
>
> It's easy to forget posture, so establish some cues: e.g. every time you check your phone, grow tall before opening the app. Studies have found people check their phone 60–80 times per day. So that means that in as little as 38–50 days, you could change your posture simply by being aware each time you check your phone. Every time you check your email 'grow tall' in your seat (email checking also adds up to typically 30–50 times per day).

3. Use your regular walks

If there is a walk you do regularly (walking to the bus stop, train station, car park, coffee shop), calculate the number of minutes it takes to get there. People take approximately 100 steps every minute they walk. If you are conscious of 'being tall' during a five-minute walk, it will account for 500 reps, meaning you can achieve good walking posture in as little as six days. On your walk, you may use your reflection in shopfronts and mirrors as more cues.

4. Wearable devices

Wearable tech such as fitness trackers can become a reminder system. If your tracker turns on/off randomly with the movement then it becomes a cue. Using this method alone can help you achieve good posture in about 100 days.

5. Sitting

Following are the most important guidelines for sitting in the right posture:

- Whenever possible, sit only in chairs with straight backs or those that support the lower back
- Always try to keep your knees a bit higher than your hips
- When sitting at an odd level, use a low stool to keep your feet on a flat surface
- When you must move while sitting, turn by moving your whole body instead of twisting your waist
- Sit straight and move your seat forward while driving. Keep a small pillow behind your lower back when going for more prolonged durations.

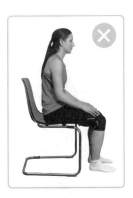 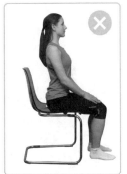 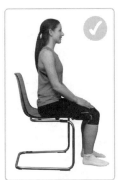

6. Standing

Follow these simple guidelines for correct standing posture to avoid damage to your lower back:

- Rest one foot on a low stool when standing for longer durations and switch the resting foot every 5–10 minutes
- Follow the standard mandate of a good standing posture, with your ears, shoulders and hips in a straight line, besides keeping your head up
- If you are in a profession where you must stand for many hours, you must stand on a surface that supports you. Surfaces like thick rubber mats always help 'absorb' the heaviness of your body. A softer texture also creates micro-movements called 'perturbations'. Perturbations help keep the body moving ever so slightly, thus reducing tension in the body. Remember, our bodies are 70% fluid encased in the softest of 'shells' called skin. Movement is part of us.

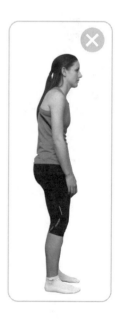 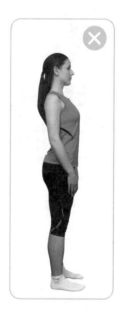 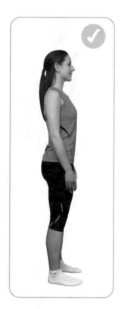

Sleeping

Sleeping on your side with knees bent is the best posture, yet there are additional guidelines that can be of immense help, which include the following:

- Use a pillow to support your neck
- Keep a pillow under your knees and another small one under the lower back, especially if you sleep on your back
- Always use a less than an eight- to ten-year-old mattress unless they have a more extended warranty period.

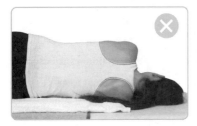 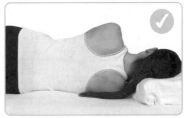

How do you know if you need a new mattress?

If you wake up in the morning feeling stiff, tight or having back pain, then try the following:

1 Sleep on another bed in the house which has a newer mattress. If you wake up feeling more refreshed without your regular mattress's aches and pains, then there is a high chance you may need to change it.

2 Sleep on a carpeted floor with 2–3 blankets as your base. Once again, if you wake up feeling better, it is time to change your old mattress.

Many come to the clinic and say, 'Kusal, I spent thousands of dollars on my current mattress. It feels fine'. My answer is always as follows: Mattress age is not necessarily an issue, and many people I have treated have had mattresses for over 15 years (actually, one couple had theirs for 24 years!) It only becomes a problem when you get back pain. In my clinical work, I have found that if the person cannot get the proper bed support after their back pain, their bodies are slower to heal, hindering the healing process.

The Research

A San Francisco University[1] study found that adopting a more upright, healthy body posture can improve mood and energy levels. The study also found that a slouched or poor body posture can lead to 'feelings of depression or decreased energy'.

Social psychologist Amy Cuddy[2], a professor and researcher at Harvard Business School, takes it one step further. Her research shows that just adopting high power or low power poses for two minutes has a measured hormonal effect.

Dr Cuddy's research found that high power poses—good, strong posture—lead to higher testosterone and link to higher confidence levels. High power poses also lower the 'stress hormone' cortisol.

The opposite is also true: adopting a low power posture leads to lower testosterone levels and higher cortisol. Dr Cuddy claims that only two minutes of high power pose is enough to make you feel more assertive and confident.

[1]Riley, P., 2012. *Research on posture yields insight into treating depression | SF State News.* [online] News.sfsu.edu. Available at: <https://news.sfsu.edu/research-posture-yields-insight-treating-depression> [Accessed 20 August 2021].

[2]Cuddy, A., 2021. *Your body language may shape who you are.* [online] Youtube.com. Available at: <https://www.youtube.com/watch?v=Ks-_Mh1QhMc&ab_channel=TED> [Accessed 20 August 2021].

The Work from Home Essentials

Unfortunately, sitting postures and sedentary lifestyles can cause a myriad of problems to the body. Our research has shown that 15 minutes of looking down at our phones (with our head down, rounded shoulders and curved upper back) is enough to cause muscle fatigue (through the spine and even arms and legs).

Muscle fatigue leads to incorrect movement patterns (you have to compensate for the fatigue somehow). These incorrect movement patterns lead to a higher chance of injury, which causes pain.

One of the side effects of this higher chance of injury is mood changes. We become lethargic, lose focus, our concentration decreases, we become more agitated and our levels of happiness drop. Overall mental wellness starts to decline. All this by working from home!

Physiotherapists closely look at a person's 24-hour cycle, which we break into three periods:

- 8 hours of Sleep (ideally!)
- 8 hours of Work
- 8 hours of Rest / Play / Recreation / Sports / Hobbies / Travel & Transit

Pre COVID-19, everyone had two things that helped them daily:

- Routine: people had a schedule for work, gym, holidays, rest, weekend, recreation, sport, family time, etc.
- Ergonomics: companies spent millions helping people get a suitable set up, correct chair, proper desks, computer screens etc.

Unfortunately, now, everything is mixed up. Routines are out the window and working from home (WFH) pretty much means working on the couch, bed, home desk whilst your partner may be doing the same thing from another room, etc. So, what can you do to get some normality back? Is normality even possible? YES! Here are some steps and tips.

Create a new routine for activity and keep this simple: Integrate exercise into your day. Create three daily exercise timeslots with an activity you love doing: morning, noon and afternoon, 30 minutes in each block.

What are the choices?

- Stretching and Flexibility
- Strength and Conditioning
- Fitness
- Fun and Family

So, what does this look like?

9am: Yoga, Pilates or Tai Chi

12 noon: Body Weight Exercises, Home Gym

3pm: Fitness using HIIT (High-Intensity Interval Training), Dancing (yes, dancing is perfect—it's fun, it involves partners, kids and family, and will improve your mood)

The key to this working for you

KEEP MOVING: NO sitting for more than 45 minutes. Seventy per cent of our composition is water—so we were meant to move. The mantra 'Any movement is an improvement' is perfect for this period.

How do you know when to move?

The body goes through three phases when we sit for an extended period:

PHASE 1: Everything feels ok. You are moving well (you have probably just sat down). You are in the GREEN ZONE.

PHASE 2: You start feeling tightness in different areas of the body—your lower back, neck, shoulders. You are now in the YELLOW ZONE.

PHASE 3: This is where the pain starts. The pain usually occurs in the lower back, moving down the leg (sciatica). You may get neck pain, headaches and shoulder pains. Also, you may aggravate pain from old injuries. That old knee injury can feel flared up, tennis elbow pain seems more sensitive, or that old RSI issue in the wrist may worsen. Now you are in the RED ZONE.

So when should you start moving? When you are in the YELLOW ZONE, stiffness and tightness is the body's way of saying 'please move'. Traditionally we have tended to ignore this warning signal from our body. When working at home, you have to be very mindful of this warning system. When you notice the stiffness, even a two-minute walk around the house, garden or even gentle stretches can make a difference for you.

Other common questions

What is the best time of the day to exercise?

There is no perfect time. The mantra is 'The Best time to exercise is WHEN you exercise'. Everybody's body clock is different. Everyone is going through various stresses—work, family, etc. so create a routine for yourself and stick to it.

What are some ways to engage the family and children?

Keep it light, make it fun and use apps, computer games, and online material. For example, create TikTok videos for fun. You choreograph a simple 10-second routine that could take the kids hours! There are myriads of online exercise classes, kids yoga, kids dancing and computer games to keep active.

How do I avoid exercise procrastination?

Put out your exercise clothes the night before. Lay them out for the kids too. Wearing workout gear will help keep you in a routine, and even if you miss a session (and you're not in your kit), it will be a subtle but strong reminder for you to exercise. Remember—your brain will always make an excuse not to exercise!

How do I make this a habit?

Keep your routine for 21 days straight. The longer you do it, the better it will be—it will create a healthy habit for you. Once you do it for this period, it will be harder to break. A by-product of a routine like this is that you will feel good.

Finally, good luck—this period of WFH is not easy. It may take months and even years for your body to assimilate to the new normal. However, if you get some semblance of routine back into your day, you will benefit. Your body and mind will thank you. You will feel good, feel loose, solid, and you will be able to work, care for your family and have a better mindset throughout.

The following is a Work from Home Ergonomic Assessment which is vital for you too. What is the Online Work from Home Ergonomic Assessment? Many people are unsure whether they are sitting correctly, whether their computer set up is ok, whether their desk position is healthy, whether their screen height is alright ... the list goes on.

Here are a few tips for getting your set up right:

- Make sure you are sitting well back in your seat (the more support your back has, the better)
- Make sure to rest your elbows on the armrests or the table or desk (elbows that are not supported cause shoulder and neck issues)
- Increase the height of your screen (make sure your eye line is forward, not downwards)
- Rule of Thumb: make sure you sit as if you were on a one-hour flight. Even on a short flight, you can rest your elbows on the arm rest, your back is comfortable against the seat, and the TV screen is at your eye level. Copy the positioning when you are working from home.

If you require further information, always speak to your physiotherapist.

What should I ask them, and what does the process include?

- Assessment of your potential problem areas (lower back, upper back, shoulders, knees, tennis/golfer's elbow or wrists)
- Exercises to overcome the problem areas (in our clinical practice, we have over 5,000 video exercises on an online program called Telehab®, developed by Vald Technologies. The portal allows you to have customised exercise programs to do at home). These will improve flexibility, strength, core, conditioning, balance and posture
- You can also send us your sitting posture (through our exercise portal) and we will assess this for you.

How many sessions could this take?

Most likely 2–3 sessions (spread over three weeks).

- 1st session: assess your body's problem areas. Set you up with the exercises to decrease pain and to prevent any further issues. After this session, you will send us a short video of your sitting posture and desk set up.
- 2nd session: assess, correct and improve desk set up to prevent issues. Update the exercises and provide you with information to continue improving and maintaining physical health whilst at home.
- 3rd session: fine-tune and progress your exercises, assess any other problem areas and provide you with tools and techniques to prevent pain.

Note: Working from home can be stressful. Stress impairs our thought processes, clear thinking pathways, and our decision-making capabilities. Stress can add to your back pain woes and magnify your pain. It's vital to take your problems to experts such as your physiotherapist, GP and your physicians at these times.

C) NUTRITIONAL GUIDELINES

The diet you maintain and how you consume it determines the way your body shapes out. Lower back pain is no exception to this rule and responds well to a planned and balanced dietary system.

Here, I've listed some of the essential guidelines you need to observe in the context of your daily nutritional habits to prevent and cure lower back pain.

Precautions:

- Food sensitivities often trigger LBP. Cut out any possible food allergens which may be in your diet. These may include dairy, wheat or gluten, chocolate, corn, soy, preservatives or food additives such as alfalfa sprouts and onions
- Try to incorporate as many antioxidant-rich foods into your diet as possible. Foods such as green leafy vegetables and fruits such as blueberries, cherries and pomegranates are good antioxidants
- Avoid refined foods such as white bread, pasta and sugar as much as possible
- Consume lean meats, cold-water fish and products like beans for proteins instead of red meats
- Use healthy cooking oils such as olive oil or vegetable oil
- Reduce the intake of trans-fatty acids to the maximum possible. Sources include bakery products such as cookies, crackers, cakes, onion rings, doughnuts and the like
- Avoid the intake of alcohol, tobacco and other such stimulants
- Have at least 6–8 glasses of filtered water daily
- Exercise for at least 30 minutes a day, for a minimum of five days a week.

Can you place a tick next to all of these?

I eat my main meals between 6am and 6pm □

Our metabolic rates are highest between 6am and 4pm so any meals consumed between these hours get broken up quickly. Most people tend to miss breakfast, have a small lunch and then eat a large dinner. It is the worst thing you can do for an exercising body. Eating a big breakfast, big lunch and small dinner will help you have better energy levels throughout the day.

I eat three vegetables and two fruits per day □

The more colourful the fruits and vegetables, the better they are for you.

I drink eight glasses of water per day □

Drinking two glasses of water first thing in the morning will help hydrate the system and prepare your body for food consumption. Overnight we do not get a chance to consume any fluids, so our cells are dehydrated. If you drink water instead of coffee first thing in the morning, it will hydrate the organs, especially the kidneys and liver, to function correctly. These vital organs help flush out toxins and purify our bodies. The third organ it helps is our skin. Skin removes toxins, so proper water consumption will reflect better, glowing skin.

I snack on fruits and low GI (glycaemic index) foods, not biscuits and fast food, between meals □

Eating healthy snacks between meals keeps up your energy levels, restores depleted energy levels, and better prepares your body for exercise. Eating foods with a low glycaemic index (low GI foods release energy slowly over time) allow you to feel fuller and have more power.

I eat meals prepared like my grandmother made □

Today meals have many additives and preservatives—especially ready meals bought from a store. Preparing the meals the same way our grandparents did will bode well for a healthy meal and healthy lifestyle.

Medicinal Supplements

Including healthy nutritional supplements in your diet can be an added advantage when you are prone to be affected by lower back pain. Here I've listed some of the most commonly suggested supplements, along with the specific benefit they offer:

- For decreasing inflammation: Omega-3 fatty acid
- For connective tissue support: Glucosamine/chondroitin
- For bone strength: Calcium/Vitamin D supplements

Herbal Supplements

Primarily available in pills, capsules and tablets, which are the standardised and dried extracts, or as tinctures and liquid extracts, herbal concoctions are a valuable preventive and curative measure for your lower back pain. Read on for a quick list of the most critical and beneficial herbal supplements available, along with their specific benefits:

- For antioxidant and immune support: Ginko (Ginko Biloba) extract
- For antioxidant and immune effects: Green tea (Camellia sinensis)
- For relief from pain and inflammation: Bromelain (Ananus comosus), Turmeric (Curcuma longa), Cat's claw (Uncaria tomentosa), Devil's claw (Harpagophytum procumbens)

CHAPTER 4

PHYSICAL
THERAPY

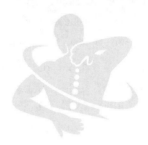

A) PHYSIOTHERAPY EXERCISE PROGRAMS

An exercise program for reducing lower back pain comprises of five categories of exercises, each having a different pre-set objective, including:

- Addressing biomechanics
- Improving mobility
- Securing quality of movement
- Core exercises
- Strength and Conditioning Exercises

Before you begin your session of exercises of lower back pain, make sure to do the following:

- Do light aerobic exercises or take a brisk walk to warm up

- Place an exercise mat or a thick blanket on the floor where you plan to exercise
- Consult your physiotherapist, GP or physician, especially if you suffer from conditions like a herniated disc.

Before you start—it's essential to understand WHY are you doing this. Here are the rules:

- **Rule 1:** Do not push past pain when you are doing exercises. Pain is a strong and intelligent indicator from your body saying that something is not correct. It lets you know your limits. Do not proceed.
- **Rule 2:** If you cannot tolerate the exercise, then you are pushing yourself too hard. Do not try and 'beat the exercise into submission'. Once again, listen to your body. Do not proceed.
- **Rule 3:** If you feel unsafe, apprehensive or unclear about an exercise then you are not ready for it. Change the activity slightly and then continue. Note the change because if you note it, then you are aware of it. If you are aware of it, you can improve from that point.
- **Rule 4:** Ensure it is ok to exercise by getting clearance from your physiotherapist, GP, or physician. If unsure, do not proceed.

The Latest Developments in Back Pain—
The Performance Pyramid

There are five fundamentals that the body needs to work at an optimum level. There is no pain, no discomfort, no apprehension with movement, or stiffness when you achieve the five fundamentals. The key fundamentals that brought the best results in the shortest period for back pain sufferers were identified by observing 50,000 treatments over 15 years.

Biomechanics

Biomechanics in the body constitutes the nerves, muscles, joints and ligaments in the body. An analysis involves looking at how they interact with a person's movement and activities as they conduct their everyday lives and their involvement in a person's behaviour. For example, stress can affect how biomechanics function, affecting a person's functional ability. The Biomechanics fundamental is the most important fundamental and is the foundation of the pyramid.

Functional Range

Once the foundation is in place, a person should be able to move. We refer to this action as their range. The range allows the person to bend forwards and backwards. If the biomechanics are not functioning well, then a person's operating or Functional Range is poor. Functional Range is the second most important fundamental.

Functional Control

Functional Control is the quality of movement. It is crucial for the smoothness of movement or action. If a person can bend forwards and touch their knees, but their activity is 'staggered' or 'step-like', they lack the quality of movement. This lack of quality means that the person's functional control is not optimum. Once the elements in the person's body are good (Biomechanics), and the person achieves their range (Functional Range), then it guarantees ease of movement (Functional Control)

Functional Core

A Functional Core is a stable base. The diaphragm, pelvic floor and a corset-like muscle—transversus abdominis work together to stabilise movement. Achieving the first three fundamentals mean getting the core correct is next in line.

Strength and Conditioning

The final fundamental is Strength and Conditioning. It is vital to maintaining the previous fundamentals. It completes the Pyramid.

The Performance Pyramid helps back pain sufferers understand which fundamentals weren't performing well and which fundamentals needed 'tweaking'. Breaking down the problem into which fundamental needs 'fixing' means a lower back pain sufferer can evaluate how much they can do themselves and when to see a practitioner. It also shows another practitioner, who they do not see as often, what areas need addressing.

The Performance Pyramid also illustrates the issue. Human beings are creatures who enjoy understanding things in a visual format. If a person understands their problem, it is easier to find ways to overcome it.

As seen in the diagram, each element has its weighting:

Biomechanics: 36.0

Functional Range: 28.0

Functional Control: 20.0

Functional Core: 12.0

Strength and Conditioning: 4.0

The weighting outlines the importance of each fundamental. As you can see, the Biomechanics is 9x more important than the Strength and Conditioning fundamental. Functional Range is 7x more important than Strength and Conditioning, and so on.
So understanding the pyramid gives LBP sufferers a clear idea of how a rehabilitation process would work.

When a person suffers from pain, many would say, 'I need to get my back stronger,' or 'I need to work on my core'. As the Performance Pyramid shows, many people only focus on the top two pyramid tiers. That means they consider a total of only 16.0 points of their problem. So many become disheartened and think that they must live with the pain. The Performance Pyramid allows them to see three more tiers (that add up to 84.0) to achieve before they feel better.

Some interesting facts about the Performance Pyramid

- For a person to feel comfortable with no back pain, they would have a total of 85.0–95.0 points. That is, each fundamental is working at 85–95% to achieve this
- If a person scores between 82–85%, they will experience apprehension and associated stiffness in their back. If a person scores between 79–81%, they will experience pain and stiffness of movement, e.g. reluctance to move with ease when getting something from the ground. Anything below 78% is pain, stiffness and apprehension
- The most important fundamental—Biomechanics—must be evaluated thoroughly by a professional experienced in assessing the condition of nerves, muscles, joints, and ligaments. To date, the most comprehensive practitioners doing this are those who follow the Ridgway Method. This method is one of the most up to date clinical reasoning processes in the world today that helps combat pain
- Once evaluated, the person can note which elements in the biomechanics their body needs to tune up regularly—for example, the tight joints in the back, gluteal tightness, or shoulder issues.

Here are the most common mistakes people make in evaluating their Performance Pyramid:

- They ignore the Biomechanics, or they get a non-professional to assess them
- They skip steps, e.g. they don't address the Functional Range, or they ignore the Functional Core fundamental
- They are impatient to progress the fundamentals to push through each fundamental without reaching an 85% score at each one, setting them back. Note: it takes approximately 4–12 weeks to work through the fundamentals.

The following diagram shows the scoring for each element. The devised scoring system provides feedback to the pain sufferer and brings attention to how much work is needed to feel better. It also requires an assessment of each fundamental, and this is usually done by a professional. However, simply understanding the five fundamentals can bring enough awareness to most to help them evaluate what is required to solve their back pain. The 21-day program follows.

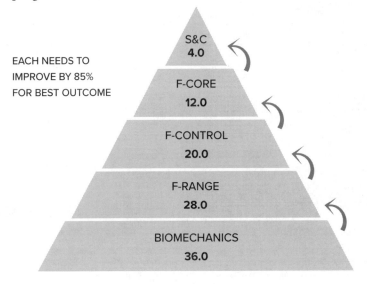

EACH NEEDS TO
IMPROVE BY 85%
FOR BEST OUTCOME

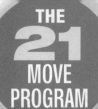

THE 21 MOVE PROGRAM

Kusal Goonewardena, Head of Sports Medicine at Elite Akademy Sports Medicine, is proud to bring you the 21 day rehab program that improves your biomechanics, mobility, control and core. It is designed to get you out of injury, reduce pain and optimise everyday movement.

	EXERCISE	1	2	3	4
FUNDAMENTAL	**Biomechanics**	Spinal Roll (20 Reps)				
		Towel Roll (10 min)				
		Gluteal Self Massage (30 sec x 3 sets)				
		Mid Back Self Massage (30 sec x 3 sets)				
	Range & Mobility	Gluteal Stretch (30 sec x 3 sets each side)				
		Piriformis Stretch (30 sec x 3 sets each side)				
		Shoulder Stretch (30 sec x 3 sets each side)				
		Hip Flexor Stretch (30 sec x 3 sets each side)				
	Control	Arm Swings (20 reps)				
		Windmill Arms (Forwards) (20 reps)				
		Windmill Arms (Backwards) (20 reps)				
		Squat Jumps (85% intensity for 30 seconds)				
		Star Jumps (85% intensity for 30 seconds)				
		Shadow Boxing (85% intensity for 30 seconds)				
	Core	Pilates Arms (1 minute)				
		Pilates Arms with Single Leg (1 minute)				
		Pilates Arms - Both Legs Up (1 minute)				
		Dead Bug (30 seconds)				
		Pilates Arms - Warm Up Routine (90 Seconds)				
		Four Point Kneel with Leg Extensions (30 sec. each leg)				
		Kneel & Lean Back (1 Minute)				
	Strength & Conditioning	As per your standard program eg. running, gym, sport, training				

NS

and complete all the highlighted exercises for that day.
to do the exercise click on the exercise to open up the video.
past pain when you do the exercises. If your pain gets worse
ately. If pain persists see your medical practitioner

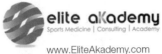

elite aKademy
Sports Medicine | Consulting | Academy

www.EliteAkademy.com
kusal@EliteAkademy.com

	7	8	9	10	11	12	13	14	15	16	17	18	19	20	21	DAY

Precautions

Remember that although a regular exercise regimen is advisable for overall fitness, specific exercises could aggravate your suffering if you overdo them. Remember to do the following activities only if you can tolerate the discomfort: football, jogging, golf, and weight training.

How do you choose a good physiotherapist and demand change in three sessions or less?

One thing separating elite athletes from the rest of us is that they demand more from their bodies—they also require more from their physios. When improvement doesn't happen quickly, elite athletes won't hesitate to seek second and third opinions from elsewhere.

In my experience, they generally expect to see a change in three sessions or less. I believe this is entirely reasonable and should inspire the rest of us. The rule of thumb is that there should be a difference in three sessions or less or a plan to achieve this. Some conditions are chronic and people may not see a change for a few months. So a good goal is paramount.

People often give too much time to treatments that are not working. In some cases, patients will remain loyal to a physio for months or years with unsatisfactory results.

I want to see the public demand more from their physiotherapists— and be prepared to seek other opinions. We should not tolerate the expense of sessions that aren't working, nor the physical discomfort endured.

As a physiotherapist, I welcome the challenge of making a difference in three sessions or less. I will gladly direct a patient elsewhere if I cannot deliver on this promise.

Patients must have high expectations and remember that not all physiotherapists are the same. Different physios will have different strengths, different knowledge and capabilities. If they fail, it doesn't mean they are no good. It usually just means a different approach is more suitable.

Expecting a positive change in three sessions or less is critical to making a fast recovery and getting back to doing what you love.

B) PILATES

'It is the mind itself that shapes the body.'
Joseph Pilates, Founder

Pilates is basically a comprehensive exercise program that encompasses the entire human body and is known to have a therapeutic effect on lower back pain.

How does it work?
Pilates works by focusing on developing the body's core strength and improving posture through a series of low impact, low repetition stretching and conditioning exercises. It works to strengthen and restore the body. Besides, Pilates also lays a strong emphasis on breathing and body awareness.

Pilates works based on six core principles, including the following:

- Centring: bringing the focus of all exercises to the centre of the body
- Concentration: promising maximum benefit if the person completes the activities with focus and commitment
- Control: especially muscle control, which should be present in each exercise
- Precision: maintained along with positioning awareness and the movement of each of the body parts in all the exercises
- Breath: integrated patterns through Pilates exercises
- Flow: that need to be maintained smoothly through each of the exercises.

C) YOGA

Yoga is widely considered one of the highly effective physical therapies to obtain relief from lower back pain. In fact, yoga can alleviate the stress associated with lower back pain to a great extent, thereby reducing the overall sensation of pain. However, experts recommend following correct instructions and consulting your physician before starting any yogic exercises, as some activities can aggravate your condition.

Here, I've briefly explained some of the most helpful yoga exercises you can perform to obtain relief from your lower back pain.

The Top 5 Yoga Workouts

1) Corpse

1 Lie flat on your back.
2 Keep your arms resting at your sides, palms down, and legs lying naturally.
3 Maintaining a relaxed position, keep your legs turned out slightly.

4 Breathe in and out slowly for a few seconds, allowing all waves of tension to escape the body.

2) Cobra pose

1 Bring yourself into the prone position.

2 Place your hands down under the shoulders.

3 Now try to raise your upper body.

4 Push the legs together if you can comfortably manage to do so.

5 In case you want a deeper stretch, you can also leave your legs slightly open.

3) Palm tree

1 Stand with your feet facing forward, arms at your sides and weight distributed on both the feet.

2 Raise your arms over your head and interlock your hands.

3 Now turn your hands in such a manner that your palms are facing upwards.

4 Place your palms on the head and turn your head, looking slightly upward.

5 Now stretch your arms upwards and come up to your toes, if it isn't painful.

6 Finally, pull your entire body upward and hold for 5–8 seconds, depending on your ability.

4) Wind-releasing pose

1 Lie flat on your back as in the Corpse pose. As you inhale in, bend your knee and place your hands right below your knee.

2 Draw your legs towards your chest.

3 Exhale and bring your forehead up to touch your knees.

4 Inhale again and now exhale as you come to your original position.

5) Fish pose

1 Lie on your back with knees bent and arms at your side.

2 Try to arch your back as far as you can do so comfortably and raise it from the ground by pushing the floor with your elbows.

3 If you can manage, tilt your head backwards and rest the crown of your head on the floor.

4 Now, breathe deeply from your diaphragm and hold for a maximum of one minute, or less if you can't manage it.

Other Activities

For the best results, combine physical exercises, yoga workouts and Pilates exercises with any combination of the following activities: walking, jogging, aerobics, biking, hydrotherapy and Tai Chi.

How to start an exercise regime that works and stick to it

The hardest part of the exercise is getting started—the next hardest is staying with it.

Thankfully, if you can stay with an exercise regime for just 28 days, then your chance of sticking with it in the long term goes through the roof. There are some things you can do to increase your chances of success dramatically. Consider the following simple secrets for establishing an exercise regime and sticking with it:

- Choose an exercise you like. Doing something you want to do, or at least can tolerate, is a critical decision in maintaining an exercise regime.
- Try not to worry too much about which is the best exercise, or what the latest fads are—any activity will be good, whether swimming, jogging, rowing, tennis, golf, cross-training or ballroom dancing. The main thing is that it's enjoyable and makes you feel good.

- Mix it up with the power of three. Mixing it up with exercise at three different intensity levels—low, medium and high intensity—is far more beneficial for your fitness and makes your exercise regime more interesting. Low-intensity exercise includes walking, gentle swimming, gardening and so on, ideally at least five days per week. Medium intensity exercise pushes you to somewhere between five-and-a-half and seven out of 10 in terms of exertion. Moderate exercise may include running, cycling, fast walking or swimming. It should be two to three times a week and for about 25–45 minutes at a time. Finally, aim for a high-intensity routine three times a week. How high is high? Push yourself to eight-and-a-half out of 10 intensity—it's just a step back from going at total capacity because any higher than this can invite injury. It is not for those with health problems and those with heart condition. If in doubt, see your doctor. High-intensity workouts can be short yet effective. I have seen great results with a three-minute training I developed, which is adaptable for anyone at any fitness level. The technique is in my book *3 Minute Workouts*.

- Buddy up. You may have friends or family members who also want to make a change—if they have a positive attitude for staying active, then you can help each other enormously. Be careful about your choice of partner—a positive partner will help you to new heights and help you stick with the routine. But a negative partner may end up draining your energy and only inspire you to give up.

- Use smart apps to stay accountable. There are many useful apps available for free on your smartphone that are great tools for keeping you accountable. Look for apps that track and rank your activity—this may require some daily inputs, but a minute or two logging your routine is worth it to track your progress and keep you engaged with your exercises. Ideally, the app will also provide you with some exercise tips.

Avoid pushing through pain. Too many fitness regimes are derailed by injury. Getting injured shouldn't stop your fitness journey, but there are a couple of critical things to remember. Number one is don't push through the pain. If while exercising you experience genuine pain, then it's time to be cautious and stop. Note, this is different from stiffness or discomfort—you may be able to work through these gently, but the pain is your body's signal to stop. If you pick up an injury, remember that recovery is possible—you may need assessment and treatment from a physiotherapist. Keep moving within tolerable pain levels while you can. Some people cease all physical activity completely when they pick up an injury. It is a mistake that may delay your recovery even more.

Mindset Tips
All exercises have a more substantial impact and better outcomes if you have a growth mindset.

CHANCES OF SUCCESS

0% I won't	60% I might
10% I can't	70% I think I can
20% I don't know how	80% I can
30% I wish I could	90% I am
40% I want to	
50% I think I might	**100% I did**

Having a solid mindset means that you can improve focus, concentrate on the path at hand to get to your goal but most importantly, enjoy the journey. Many people look at the goal but do not enjoy the steps that they are taking. If you are enjoying the process, you are more likely to achieve your exercise goals.

Can you place a tick next to all of the following?

I know yoga or Pilates and enjoyed doing some of these sessions in weekly or fortnightly classes in the past ☐

I know what meditation is and have practised this in the past ☐

I enjoy a challenge. I embrace it instead of avoiding it ☐

Coming up against obstacles makes me want to overcome them rather than losing my momentum and shying away from them ☐

What's the minimum you need to do to stay fit as you age (gracefully)?

Is there a bare minimum level of exercise that will keep you fit? It's an easy question, but the answer is more complicated.

Everyone responds differently to exercise. What works for friends or family might not work for you. Finding a handy 'one-size-fits-all' solution is challenging, yet any 'bare minimums' for exercise must involve moving often.

The giant trap for people is gradually restricting your movement. It usually happens so slowly you don't notice it. Sometimes there are genuine issues that may cause you to move a little less, whether consciously or unconsciously—for example, there might be injuries or ailments, including arthritis, which can slow you down. One thing we know for sure is lack of movement only makes these issues worse.

Even those suffering from pain or arthritis will benefit from moving regularly within tolerable pain levels. If the pain is too much, then a professional assessment and treatment are required—this should also provide a plan to increase your ability to move gradually.

Your fitness depends on many other things too—for example, your diet, whether you are a smoker or non-smoker, and how much alcohol you consume every week.

If we consider a person with a good diet, a non-smoker and a moderate drinker, the following might be viewed as the minimum to stay fit.

There's no great secret—you must be moving at least half an hour a day to have any chance of building fitness. This movement could be walking, swimming, gardening, cycling, dancing—whatever you like.

For many people, the easiest way to be sure is to walk 30 minutes a day, five days a week at least, at moderate intensity (not too slow but not power-walking). And then if you have other interests, such as gardening or swimming or golf, that's a bonus. If you're up for trying yoga or Pilates, then that would be outstanding.

The other very important thing to add is trying to avoid sitting down too much at any one time. It's essential to get up and about regularly to keep your joints, ligaments and muscles in good shape.

I would also add this brings up an interesting philosophical question. Is living a happy and healthy life just about doing the bare minimum, or can it be more than that? What are the benefits of doing a little bit more?

I would argue that going beyond the bare minimum has enormous benefits for physical and mental wellbeing. And research backs me up on this, with several highly regarded studies espousing the benefits of incorporating higher intensity exercises into the mix.

My minimum involves exercise at low, medium and high intensities. Remember that low-intensity exercise can be walking, gentle swimming, gardening and so on for a minimum of 30 minutes at least five days per week. Medium intensity exercise pushes you a little more, with an effort between 5.5 and seven out of ten, two to three times a week for about 25–45 minutes each time is ideal.

High-intensity exercise is where you ramp it up to an 8.5 out of ten effort. It's not for everyone, and it's recommended you see a health professional first if you are unsure. A high-intensity burst of even 1–2 minutes, three times a week, can give you that fitness edge.

The myths about stretching debunked

For some reason, there's an ongoing debate about whether to stretch or not before exercise. With so many opinions, it must seem challenging to know what is right for you. But in over 20 years' practice in physiotherapy, my opinion has never wavered— stretching was, is, and will always be necessary for your general bodily maintenance, especially before exercise and sports. I have encountered many myths around stretching—here are some doozies you may have heard:

Myth: Stretching alone can prevent injury

If only it were that simple. Unfortunately, there's no guarantee stretching can prevent injury. There are too many variables at play: muscles can be weak, joints can be stiff or too loose, nerves can be tight, ligaments strained. Any of these alone or together can cause injury.

Stretching works wonders for tight muscles, but there are plenty of other issues that can go wrong, and stretching won't necessarily prevent your joints, nerves, or ligaments. If you are stretching yet repeatedly becoming injured, you may need a professional assessment to find exactly where you are breaking down.

Myth: If you're inflexible, then stretching is important

Many issues cause Inflexibility, not just tight muscles. Even stress and incorrect diet can cause inflexibility. Stretching is not the only solution, though it is likely to be useful for you. But if you have ongoing issues with flexibility, you may need a professional assessment to evaluate your muscles, joints, nerves, and ligaments.

Myth: If you're already flexible, you're okay!

Unfortunately, this is not only untrue but believing this may contribute to future injuries.

If you're flexible, you still need to prepare your muscles for activity. I would still recommend starting with static stretches (just a basic stretch for about 30 seconds) and then working up to dynamic stretches (more functional stretches where your joints and muscles go through complete movements).

Myth: If you don't stretch, your muscles will shorten

Incorrect. Muscles will only shorten if kept in a compressed (closed) position. For example, always having your arm bent will shorten your biceps muscle. But you could go all your life using your arm, without stretching your biceps, and not worry.

What are some keys to an excellent stretching routine?

Creating a stretching routine is good—you loosen your body gradually before activity. Note: you shouldn't feel pain. If you're feeling pain, you are pushing yourself too much.

Beware of pins and needles or numbness when stretching. They occur by pushing the nerves or biomechanical structures past what they can tolerate. Again, you need to ease off.

When you are stretching, hold the stretch for 30 seconds—research says 21 seconds is enough, but 30 seconds is a nice round number, and those extra nine seconds won't hurt.

Repeat the stretch on each muscle three times before moving onto another muscle.

Opinions vary on whether to stretch your upper or lower body first. It depends on the exercise you are doing. Swimming is mainly an upper body workout, so it's always good to stretch the upper body first and then move to lower limbs. For runners or other exercises which mainly uses the lower body, it's vice versa—stretch the lower limbs first, then move to the upper body. Many people tend to chop and change—upper body first on one occasion, lower body another—this is not as effective.

Stretching the upper back and lower back is vital for any exercise—

gentle twisting, turning and bending stretches are effective. Static stretching, which is a basic muscle stretch for 30 seconds, is suitable for everyday maintenance.

Dynamic stretches are good before an activity which means that you may mimic an action, for example, moving your leg in a pendulum-like fashion. These actions let the muscles stretch, create movement through the joints, and increase blood flow to the area.

While stretching should be a part of the warm-up, stretching should not be the sole warm-up. Research has shown this to be true. Remember to ease into any exercise you are doing.

D) HYDRATION, COMPRESSION WEAR AND RECOVERY: YOUR TOOL KIT FOR SUCCESS

I am building a fire, and every day I train, I add more fuel.
At just the right moment, I light the match.
Mia Hamm

The world of exercise is indeed an enigmatic arena. It is a juncture where the ideal amalgamation of human sentiment, strength and endurance is on an intense display. The Zen is to make it work and strike a chord of completion, which results in pain relief, and a solid performance pyramid.

Those who persevere long after the others might have quit or changed tracks are the ones who finally achieve the pinnacle. Your path. Your choice!

So what makes all the difference?

It has all to do with the path you choose.

It has all to do with how you set your goals.

It has all to do with the way you plan your success.

And finally, it has everything to do with your tools, aides and guides,

your companions on the path to hard work and success.

Read on to explore the fantastic world of some of the best tools you can take with you on this beautiful journey!

Success, we now know, is all unison of intelligent planning, sharp focus, a clear vision and lots of labour. Funnily enough, when you have the first three down pat, the 'labour' is not bad. Things are even more enjoyable.

Many people see analysis and effort as two different fields of study in the world of back pain rehabilitation. Sometimes even for an active person it is often not viable or even possible to gauge the extent to which their choices and visions will make a difference. Both sides of the equation are, however, equally important.

While the niche of analysis, study and research always righteously rested with the vast diasporas of analysts and research scientists, so the vision and wisdom of a coach and guide determine the rehabilitation course's outcomes. It is true even for the best out there. The tools you choose actually become your partners in success and glory.

Here I want to highlight the relevance and critical importance of three beneficial tools that you can use in back pain rehabilitation.

In the following pages, you will find detailed sections on each of these aspects: Hydration, Compression wear and Time for Recovery.

Hydration encompasses the entire study of concepts such as dehydration, sports drinks and alcohol abuse.

Compression wear, including its relevance, the right choice of such gear and the best ways to make use of it.

Time for Recovery, including boosting back performance and the value of fast-tracking back pain rehabilitation.

As you read on, you will realise that it is quite a fantastic journey into how each of these aspects, successfully managed, achieves an optimum rehab level for your back pain.

Take each tool as a separate, isolated aspect of analysis. Attempt to understand each tool in its own light. Begin by analysing your road of rehabilitation and make an effort to correlate how one or more of these three aspects can help you achieve more.

Knowledge is Empowerment!

In most science and logic fields, there is technical jargon used instead of common terminology. The trend makes language complicated and more demanding for everyday people to understand. Also, over-using technical jargon in common vocabulary might take away its original meaning. So, even the best out there might be unaware of what some of these terms mean. Complicating language can adversely affect the output of a person in their respective field. So, to begin with, let's unravel language and look at what the term 'performance' actually implies in a specific context to back pain rehabilitation.

Performance—An Analysis

Active movements are considered a physical activity in which the patient or client applies their motor reflexes to propel their bodily movements to achieve a pre-defined target. Simply put, performance is the measure of how well the motor reflexes move in the context of these pre-set goals.

In specific industrial terminology, performance is the act of carrying out specific, well-defined physical routines and procedures by an individual trained in physical activity. It is indeed a competitive world out there. In physiological terms, there is ongoing strife between the body, mind, and soul to get the better of each other. In the pursuit of higher accomplishments and achievements, we are constantly searching for what helps our body improve. At the same time, we also tend to eye the critical roadblocks to see what might be preventing our body from performing to its best. If we want to understand the significance and impact of a particular field of study, we must look at each minuscule aspect from a macro perspective. It is crucial if we want to achieve perfection and excellence in a discipline.

First, let us begin by understanding more about performance as it is the most important term and concept in back pain rehabilitation. Performance brings the entire physical and psychological setup of our knowledge into action. Here, the human mind and body are inter-connected through a series of physiological and behavioural mechanisms.

It is a common misconception that an individual's performance in physical activity or well-being results from physical strength, stamina, or ability. In fact, it is an inter-connected mechanism at work. Let us look at this phenomenon in detail before learning about what elements make a difference in back pain rehabilitation.

The Mind-Body Connection

In back pain, 90 per cent of performance is mental.

In a world where most of our efforts only improve our

physical training, this fact can indeed change the way we look at rehabilitation and performance. On the conscious level, it is the physical network of muscles, joints, ligaments and tendons that propel the person forward. However, the contrary might be very accurate.

The conscious and subconscious mind hugely influence our core logic. How our mind affects our performance in well-being and other activities we think lies in the principle that the conscious mind is at the forefront of our mental makeup. It is the front end of our mind. In our everyday activities, we are aware of the conscious mind. However, our subconscious mind is the key driving force behind the conscious mind. The subconscious mind programs our conscious mind to behave the way it does. It is the back-end of the mind, and it is vitally essential for the front end to perform well. Funnily enough, both work hand in hand, and without the subconscious other efforts become invalid for the back pain sufferer.

Those faithful to the back pain rehabilitation process find a critical connection between the body and the mind. It is a proven fact that the mind controls the human body. It is firstly vital to train and attune the mind if we want to drive the body effectively.

Hard-core training of a person indeed starts with mental conditioning and neuromuscular control exercises. It is almost impossible to achieve a perfect level of training and excellence in well-being without conditioning the mind to be balanced, positive and focused. Some studies demonstrate demarcated success and lack of success of people in the spinal rehabilitation process using specific personality structure and mood state measures.

Apart from the basic understanding of mind over the body and post-performance, another exciting fact emerges in this context.

According to specific findings made by the famous neurobiologist Fred H. Gage the rate of generating new cells and brain activity is strongly influenced by the individual's interaction with the environment. As is evident, regular, rigorous exercise is one of the best ways of interacting with the environment.

The Role

So, how exactly does the mind influence our body in the specific context of performance? Well, in activity, there are goals and training targets to be met. Most often, these goals are higher in proportion to the person's capability. The person has to be mentally strong enough to look within themselves and spot their drawbacks and the weaker zones that might be stopping them from reaching their goals if they want to achieve these targets.

Equipped with this clarity of mind, someone skilled in this understanding can then effectively work towards gaining mobility, control, strength and improving themselves in the aspects required. It is one of the critical ways the mind exercises a crucial influence over the body to perform. In fact, it is often the mental distraction at the time of performance that is one of the top reasons for lack of achievement. Dr Kristen Race, PhD and founder of Mindful Life, tells us, 'When our brains get caught up in thoughts of the future or the past, we can't use the part of the brain that keeps us engaged at the moment,' and this mental chatter can make it very difficult for the regular person to focus and achieve their goal.

Take a Step

In your pursuit to achieve perfection in back pain rehabilitation, your first step ought to be to gain control of your mind or at least understand its mannerisms. A person who succeeds in rehab is one who eventually learns to master the mechanics of their mind. If they achieve this, they can then learn to drive their physical efforts by the sheer force of their mental strength.

Here, it is interesting to know how every person can reach the peak in their chosen activity, hobby or sport. The key lies in the person's ability to identify their strengths, weaknesses and the key obstacles in their way to peak performance. The barriers disappear once the real power of the mind is there.

Factors that Matter

There is a vast range of factors that influence an individual's performance in both outdoor and indoor activities. From physical strength, stamina and previous medical history to aspects like genetics, nutrition and lifestyle, all these factors go a long way in determining the primary performance of a person's back pain rehabilitation. Several methods can explain these factors. However, it is advisable to study them in an organised and structured manner. In this section, we shall enlist the key performance factors that determine the level of performance in rehab.

Physical Ability and Strength

Physical ability and strength are the topmost determinants of the quality of performance. These factors encompass a broad range of aspects of physical ability. Some of the elements are:

- Physical strength and stamina
- Endurance levels
- Level of agility and flexibility
- Quality of neuromuscular coordination
- Basic body type

Health History

A person's previous medical history and present status play a significant role in determining levels of performance. The risks for poor performance are high if the individual suffers from even minor cardiovascular, respiratory or orthopaedic issues.

Genetics

It is interesting to know that genetics make a difference in what kind of a person you eventually become. If your lifestyle and other factors are in place, your genes can go a long way in determining your muscle size, physical strengths, and muscle fibre composition. In addition, genetics can influence the anaerobic threshold (AT), lung capacity, and so on. But good genes are not a reflection of the talent and, finally, the outcome. In short, those who don't have the best gene pool can still achieve whatever they put their mind to.

Nutrition

People recovering from back pain need to have a specially designed diet plan to provide them with enough energy before, during and after exercises. The power required goes into the healing process.

Equipment and Gear

The equipment and gear used also determines the quality of improvement. In fact, these are the tools for a person undergoing back pain rehab, and it is vital to pay adequate attention to these aspects. Towards this end, we shall study more about compression wear.

Personality Traits

Every person has a different personality structure. However, some factors are imperative for all those who want to succeed. They include high motivation, a sense of discipline, a balanced temperament, and so on. The absence of any such factors can harm the level of a rehab success.

Lifestyle

Stimulants like alcohol and cigarette smoking can negatively impact the quality of performance in back pain rehabilitation. In addition, lifestyle factors like a disciplined routine and regulated sleep quality, as already discussed, also make a difference.

The 3 Key Tools—A Preamble

The field of back pain rehabilitation is indeed a vast sphere of study. It is an unimaginable blend of intense physical stamina, mental strength and emotional grit.

As we just studied, it is virtually impossible to account for or even look at all the possible factors that could ever influence an individual's rehab journey. After all, everyone has a different body constitution and varied strengths and weaker zones. Psychologists and analysts have always mulled over innovative ways to enhance the existing levels of output amongst people. For this study, this section of the book deals with three such essential aspects that can contribute to success in back pain rehabilitation.

Hydration

In the following sections, you will realise how hydration plays a crucial role in determining the efficiency level of a person going through this journey. You will read about the benefits of staying adequately hydrated and the loss of efficiency due to dehydration. As you read on, you will also know about some of the most harmful effects of alcohol. Finally, you will learn some valuable facts about electrolyte supplements and energy drinks.

Compression Wear

Compression garments are one of the most valuable tools when it comes to improvement in performance levels. You will learn more about how such compression wear helps enhance overall efficiency, reduces injuries, and finally, plays a significant role in improving the overall quality of movement, thus fast-tracking the rehabilitation process.

Recovery

This book effectively explains how proper recovery is vital for improving performance and the prevention of injury including looking at a series of healing methods such as massage, contrast baths and much more.

HYDRATION—THE LIFELINE

Key Definitions

Water is the vital life force of human existence. The body has its own systematic ways of maintaining the right amounts of these essential nutrients in its system. Hydration, as a term, encompasses the entire gambit of processes and actions by which fluid is input into the body.

Hydration

A definition of hydration is the process by which the human body ingests and absorbs water. The hydration process possesses critical importance since water plays a vital role in a series of bodily functions. Staying duly hydrated is seen as one of the most critical factors that can impact the level of performance and rehab.

What is Dehydration?

Dehydration is typically the state where the human body cannot effectively cool itself. Experts define dehydration as the dynamic loss of body water, causing severe health consequences.

The Hydration Balance

As with various other aspects of sports and fitness, there is no exact and generic limit to the amount of water that people should consume. The limit might vary according to the individual, their body constitution and the type of activity they are undergoing. Nevertheless, an understanding exists for the amount of water consumed before, during, and after exercise. Many experts then lay down a generic range of water people should have before, during and after their activity. These vary around the world.

Please refer to the chart below for a sample guideline.

STAGE OF EXERCISE	AMOUNT OF WATER	TIME OF CONSUMPTION
Before exercise	500ml	2–3 hours before starting
Before exercise	250ml	20–30 minutes before starting
During exercise	250ml	Every 10–20 minutes during exercise
After exercise	250ml	After 30 minutes

A Good Rule of Thumb

Athletes can measure the amount of fluid they lose during exercise to help them ascertain how much water their body needs to stay properly hydrated. Technically, one needs to consume 500ml for every 500 grams they lose during exercise. They have sweated, burnt, used up this much water from their bodies. Another mode of rehydrating is to continue drinking water until your urine colour turns from yellow/ orange to a clear or straw colour. When the body is dehydrated, the colour of your urine is yellow to orange.

Causes of Dehydration

Before we go on about the benefits of hydration, causes of dehydration and ways to keep yourself hydrated first, how does our body lose moisture in the first place?

When we exercise, our core body temperature rises above its usual level or range. When this level increases, our bodily systems come into action and try to lower the temperature or cool it down. The most important method by which the body attempts to cool itself is through sweating. So, if equal or more amounts of fluids do not replace the amount of water lost during such sweating, the body becomes dehydrated.

Research shows that a session of intense physical exercise can cause our body to lose as much as 1.0–2.5 L of fluids in the form of sweat per hour. In this case, dehydration will occur if we do not maintain the level of intake of fluids.

Experts point out a vast range of causes of dehydration. In this section, I've briefly listed the most important causes of dehydration.

- Prolonged hours of physical activity without an adequate intake of fluids is the most common cause of dehydration. When your body begins to lose a greater amount of sweat than you have replenished, dehydration would definitely occur.

- Absence of specially formulated hydration drinks also accounts for higher levels of dehydration. When you do not consume enough electrolytes to compensate for the loss of vital nutrients, your body is likely to become dehydrated.

- Excessive clothing and improper gear can also be another cause of dehydration. Sportswear should ideally be made of natural fabrics that allow the skin and body to breathe well. There will be more about compression wear, one such component of clothing to wear when exercising, in the coming pages.

- Some people also complain of dehydration after a sudden increase in the duration and intensity of physical exercise. In such cases, the body cannot cope with the massive loss of fluids and hence begins to show the signs of dehydration.

- Exercising in sweltering and humid weather can also cause rapid water loss from the body, thus causing dehydration.

The Performance Booster—Top 7 Benefits

Water is indeed the true elixir of life. To stay hydrated is not a conscious choice you make. It is not a luxury you can have or leave. Instead, it is necessary. It is an inevitable step you must take to enhance your sporting performance to the optimum level.

The human body is 70% water. With 70% of the earth also comprising water, it is indeed the true-life force of human existence. In fact, water, when had in quantity, at the right time, can be one of the most vital reasons for good health and excellent performance in rehab.

Experts strongly emphasise that proper hydration is an important part of the preparation, recovery, and participation of every person, especially in competitive settings.

Though it is a vast subject of study and analysis, I have listed some of the most crucial and vital benefits of staying hydrated, especially for everyday people. You will also read about how water is crucial for various bodily functions, apart from boosting the overall performance. Read on for the top seven reasons why you need to watch your hydration levels at all costs.

It is a cooling agent

Water is the top form of hydration for people. Experts warn that after a certain limit of moisture loss, supplementation with energy drinks and electrolytes becomes important, yet water remains the primary cooling and hydrating agent.

Strength and endurance

Proper hydration goes a long way in ensuring high-performance levels by increasing overall levels of strength and endurance. People who are properly hydrated most of the time are likely to have better stamina, focus and clarity of their goals.

It regulates the thermoregulatory system

The body's thermoregulatory system is the mechanism by which the body regulates its internal temperature through various interconnected processes in the brain, liver and cardiovascular systems. Blood plasma, which is the fluid component of blood, is 90% water. When there is a loss of water from the body, it makes the blood thicker and less efficient to move within the blood vessels, carrying oxygen and other vital nutrients.

It helps in the regulation of cortisol levels

Research shows that a lower level of hydration in the body leads to increased production of the cortisol hormone, also known as the stress hormone. Higher levels of cortisol can cause extreme mental stress, anxiety and even depression in a person.

It helps maintain body weight

Adequate hydration is required to replace the loss of fluid from the body during physical exercise. When there is a wide gap between the amount of fluid lost and replaced, it often results in unnecessary loss of the person's body weight.

It helps regulate critical bodily functions

Water plays a vital role in regulating a series of bodily functions. Here are a few essential points about some of the most critical bodily functions relevant to adequate hydration:

- Transportation of nutrients and oxygen to body cells
- Improving blood circulation
- Helping in the regeneration of new cells
- Moistening the mucous membrane
- Helping in cushioning and lubricating the joints
- Helping in converting food into the required amount of energy
- Assisting in the removal of waste material from the body
- Aiding in the absorption of vital nutrients.

It aides recovery

Adequate hydration is crucial for better recovery from the stress and fatigue of exercise.

6 Key Signs of Dehydration

General fatigue is the first and most prominent sign of dehydration. However, since fatigue can also occur due to various other reasons such as excessive exertion or illness, the signals are often overlooked. It is vital for the person and the allied health team supporting them to be alert for any of these signs to avoid any severe consequences.

In this section, we have laid down some of the most important signs of dehydration.

Dizziness

When dehydrated, you will start feeling dizzy or light-headed. In the beginning, this sensation might appear to be a result of general fatigue. However, if this continues for a more extended period, it is a definite sign of dehydration and should be put to rights immediately.

Nausea

A person who is feeling dehydrated will have frequent spells of nausea. They will have a repetitive urge to vomit, even though they might not have eaten anything for a while. Such episodes of nausea are incredibly intense while exercising.

Dryness in the mouth

A dehydrated person is often licking their lips due to dryness. It mainly happens when exercising in hot conditions. The mouth, tongue and lips will feel parched. The ideal way to avoid dehydration in hot and humid conditions is to drink smaller quantities of water after short intervals.

Increased heartbeat

A person who has not been taking enough fluids will experience a very high rate of beats per minute (BPM). They must inform the physiotherapist, GP or physician immediately if the heartbeat doesn't return to resting levels.

Cramped and tired muscles

If your muscles are getting tight and achy consider whether it could be dehydration. The sensation is quite different from feeling tired or exhausted. There are intense cramps in muscles even after a slight amount of over exertion.

Minimal sweating

A person who drinks less water will sweat less. If you have finished a round of intense workout in hot or humid conditions and are still not sweating, it could be a sign of dehydration.

Some of the other signs include:

- Reduced level of endurance
- Slower muscular response
- Abnormal loss in body weight
- Improper functioning of the kidneys
- Wrong working of the digestive system

Interestingly, even a 2% loss of water from the body can trigger the onset of the above symptoms in a person.

Illnesses and consequences

When a person is dehydrated, they can experience mild to severe illness, depending on the intensity of the problem.

Below, I briefly discuss each of the possible outcomes of dehydration, including the conditions it can eventually cause.

Mild dehydration—Heat cramps

In this case, the body of a dehydrated person will not be able to cool itself in humid conditions. When the process of dehydration starts, the individual is just likely to experience painful cramps, also known as heat cramps.

The most prominent symptoms of heat cramps will be excruciating spasms in the stomach, legs, arms, and back muscles.

Mild to moderate dehydration—Heat exhaustion

The symptoms of heat exhaustion are more prominent and often severe. If a person is facing excessive dehydration, they will likely experience the following symptoms of heat exhaustion:

- Weakness or lack of strength in legs
- Extreme nausea
- Severe headache
- High heartbeat per minute (BPM) or pulse rate
- Low blood pressure

Severe dehydration—Heatstroke

Heatstroke is the most severe outcome of dehydration. It is also known as the most severe form of heat-related illnesses. In fact, it can even prove fatal if left untreated.

Some of the prominent signs include:

- High body temperature, usually above 40°C or 104°F
- High BPM
- Hot skin flushes

- The quickened pace of breathing
- Loss of consciousness
- Delirium and hallucinations
- Seizures

Hydration Drinks

Water is usually considered the best form of fluid for people. However, when the volume and intensity of physical exercise increase beyond a limit, it is virtually impossible to stay duly hydrated without adequate supplementation.

In ideal conditions, sports drinks need to have at least 8% carbohydrate content to boost the rate of water absorption and improve overall performance. The sports drink industry has diversified to a considerable extent, and the options available for supplementation are vast. Each form of hydration drink has its pros and cons. We will discuss two popular forms of supplements in this section for analytic study, namely Energy Drinks and Electrolytes. Read on for a brief description of both and to know which is the more preferred one.

Energy Drinks

Energy drinks are a category of carbonated hydration drinks comprising stimulants such as caffeine and sugar, meant to give an immediate energy boost, especially for sportspersons. The critical aim of energy drinks is to boost mental and physical energy, though they usually work only in a shorter period.

Energy drinks have been quite popular in the last few decades, especially amongst youngsters and the non-professional sporting types. The main reason is the immediate energy boost and refreshing flavour or differing taste. However, in the last few years, this form of hydration drinks has earned bad press due to various reasons.

Research shows that over-consumption of energy drinks can often lead to severe consequences such as:

- Irritability
- Insomnia
- Nervousness
- Allergic reactions
- Increased heartbeat per minute (BPM)
- High blood pressure

Despite the above-reported side effects, energy drinks are still used extensively in the world of activity and sport. A report said that even in the face of the increased FDA scrutiny of the safety of these energy drinks, the drink sales went up by 6.7% in the USA in the year 2013 alone.

Some of the most famous brands of energy drinks include Monster, Red Bull, Rockstar, NOS, Full Throttle, Amp, Rip It, Venom, Arizona Energy and Xyience Xenergy.

Electrolyte Supplement Drinks

An electrolyte is an umbrella term given to the group of vital nutrients required by the human body, including potassium, sodium and magnesium. Each of these nutrients gets lost to a great extent through sweat, the natural cooling mechanism of the human body. Electrolyte drinks should offer enough replacement for the loss of these nutrients. Some of the most well-known and effective electrolyte drinks include Powerade, Gatorade and All Sport.

Research shows how some of the most prominent signs of

dehydration are direct consequences of losing electrolytes from the body. These symptoms include severe muscle cramps and side stitches. Understanding how electrolyte drinks benefit your body, it is first essential to know the constituents of electrolytes. As an element, electrolytes primarily consist of the following components:

- Calcium (Ca 2+)
- Sodium (Na+)
- Potassium (K+)
- Magnesium (Mg 2+)
- Chloride (Cl-)
- Phosphate (PO4 2-)
- Bicarbonate (HCO3-)
- Sulfate (SO4 2-)

The signs of + and − with each of the above constituents indicate that these minerals are ionic. The ionic nature gives the electrolytes the power to carry electrical energy that helps the proper functioning of the body's systems. Amongst the above, the first four electrolytes are the most important. They help in maintaining the basic fluid balance in the body.

The Ingredients

A healthy electrolyte drink should ideally have the following ingredients (per 250ml), though the proportion can vary slightly:

- Carbohydrates, 14 g
- Potassium, 28 mg
- Sodium, 100 mg

Know Your Choices—The Electrolyte Logic

When it comes to comparison, experts strongly vouch for the efficacy of electrolyte drinks in the long run rather than energy drinks. Let's understand the underlying logic here.

Scientists point out an intriguing logic explaining the importance of electrolytes. By now, we know how important it is to maintain a proper intake of fluids and water before, during and after exercise to stay properly hydrated. However, it is a little known fact that you still might not get proper hydration even after you have consumed the right amounts of water, if electrolytes are missing in your fluid intake. So, what is the underlying logic?

The Reason

1. Loss of Minerals

When you sweat, your body just doesn't lose water. It also loses significant amounts of minerals, including sodium, magnesium, potassium and calcium. You will stay dehydrated unless you supplement your fluid intake with an adequate amount of these electrolyte drinks.

Sodium

Amongst these four minerals, your body loses the maximum amount of sodium during intense physical activity. Hence, an electrolyte drink should ideally contain high proportions of this particular mineral.

Potassium

Similarly, potassium is a mineral that allows the movement of nutrients and fluids across the cells of your body. In turn, it enables the cells to move ahead with their regular metabolic functions, such as muscle contraction. In the absence of enough quantities of potassium, your muscles will be unable to generate the required nerve pulses, which regulate muscle contraction.

As is evident, the performance in activity will get seriously affected when your muscles cannot perform the required movements.

As a rule of thumb, any person indulging in intense physical activity for more than one hour needs supplementation in the form of electrolyte drinks. The most prominent symptom of electrolyte deficiency in the body is severe muscle cramping.

2. The Dilution Effect

Experts also point out another disastrous effect of inadequate intake of electrolytes. Consider a situation where there is an absence of these vital minerals listed above. If you have only plain water, in this case, you will end up diluting the concentration and effect of the remaining electrolyte minerals that still exist in your body. It will eventually impair your performance ability to a great extent.

Alcohol Abuse

Alcohol is seen as the single-most major impediment to performance and is a significant factor in slowing down the speed of back pain rehabilitation.

Recent research by the NHS in the UK over one week showed that around 55 per cent of men and 53 per cent of women drank more alcohol than the recommended guidelines. Ironically, a similar report also indicated that within the year 2014, almost 15.6 million people in the UK played some form of sport at least once a week.

Here, the irony lies in the fact that the regular over-consumption of alcohol might counteract the benefits gained from such sporting activities. Well, researchers define two straightforward ways in which alcohol mars your performance as a person who goes through rehab. Let's look at both of these reasons closely.

1. The Diuretic Effect

Alcohol is basically a diuretic in nature. It will naturally make your kidneys produce more urine, leading to dehydration in the long run. You can read about the dire consequences of dehydration in the above sections.

By now, you know your body loses so much water in the form of sweat when you exercise. This loss is further compounded by the diuretic effect, causing the body's hydration levels to drop much below the desired level. When such dehydration happens, the flow of blood is affected, which impairs its ability to transport oxygen and other nutrients across the body's cells.

2. The Energy Levels

Alcohol interferes strongly with your body's process of generating energy. Your liver needs to work much harder to break down alcohol and produce lower glucose levels. Consequently, the levels of blood sugar will fall and will lead to a drop in energy. It will, in turn, affect your performance in sports since you need higher levels of energy to perform to your best potential.

Apart from the above, there are a few other ways in which alcohol affects your performance in sports, which include:

• It reduces your overall speed, strength and stamina

- It causes excess depletion of vitamins and minerals due to increased water levels
- It slows your reaction time due to poor hand-eye coordination and overall body balance
- It depresses the immune system
- It lowers the pace of muscle recovery
- It negatively impacts your memory
- It affects your body metabolism, as the body converts alcoholic calories into fatty acids
- It can reduce the serum testosterone levels, leading to decreased lean muscle mass
- It harms the quality of your sleep
- It can cause a more significant number of muscular cramps due to an increased quantity of lactic acid
- It interferes with your ability to exercise correctly, especially when you have a hangover.

Stay Hydrated—Useful tips

- Make sure you are well hydrated before you start exercising
- Do not wait to feel thirsty during exercise. Make sure you have water at regular intervals. Refer to the chart on page 74 for the amount of water you should have before, during, and after exercise
- Always keep a watch on the colour of your urine. You might be dehydrated if your urine is excessive yellow or even orange or has a strong smell
- Make sure water is a part of every meal
- Decrease your consumption of sugary drinks
- Use marked and refillable water bottles to keep track of the amount of water you have consumed

- The choice of your drink makes a difference. Conventionally, water and fluids can be interchangeable terms for some. Experts emphasise that water is traditionally the best fluid replacement option for the human body. However, water needs to be supplemented with adequate specially formulated drinks for high-intensity physical activity. Refer to the section above for further reference

- The time you drink water also makes a difference. The chart on page 74 effectively explains the right time to have water or other drinks before and after exercise. It is essential to follow these guidelines to keep your body hydrated to the correctly required levels.

COMPRESSION WEAR—THE MIRACLE TOOL

Know the Basics

The above section of the book analysed how hydration can act as a fantastic tool for improving your performance in back pain rehab. Hydration or the lack of it can actually serve as the single most crucial factor for improving or worsening your performance in sports.

On similar lines, in this section, I shall present a detailed analysis of compression wear as a tool for increasing the outcome of rehab performance. You will read all about how using the proper compression wear can reduce the rate and intensity of pain whilst improving the overall balance and quality of movement.

Foremost, we shall begin by understanding all about the concept of compression wear.

Compression wear is a group term given to a type of close-fitting clothing made from high quality elasticised material. Traditionally, athletes wear this form of clothing to provide unique utility and comfort to the relevant muscles and body parts. Experts suggest that the main advantage of compression wear comes from its ability to improve the level of blood circulation and oxygen delivery across the body, thus implying that anyone who wants to strengthen movement can wear it.

The Logic

The logic behind the basic design of compression wear is that a better blood flow and oxygen consumption in the body achieves the following:

- It boosts performance
- It reduces the risk of injury
- It reduces fatigue levels
- It decreases pain levels
- It increases awareness due to the compression on the skin.

Compression wear design uses highly engineered, elastic gradient compression fabric. The particular material enables the garment to mould around the body with ease. Eventually, it aims to increase the blood and lymphatic flow.

The compression clothing can deliver specific and gradual levels of pressure to the relevant body part. The typical pressure exerted by such clothing ranges from 20–40 millimetres of mercury. More specifically, custom-designed compression wear delivers pressure according to medical-grade standards.

The Key Types

Read on to know more about some of the most important and popular types of compression wear.

Compression Socks and Stockings

Compression stockings work by improving the flow of blood to the legs. When you wear them, the stockings gently squeeze your legs. This action results in the movement of blood in the upward direction in your legs. You can opt for the socks and stockings in varying heights, ranging from knee-length socks to ankle socks.

Tops and T-shirts

Compression tops and t-shirts come in various fits and styles. You can opt for the full-sleeved top, the half-sleeved t-shirt or even the sleeveless upper wear, depending on your activity. These tops and t-shirts work by stabilising the muscles in sports like weight training, tennis and running.

Tights

Compression tights protect and guard the leg muscles, which are the largest muscle group in the body. These are ideal for sports such as running, cycling, football, tennis, basketball and netball.

Shorts

Compression shorts are basically a skin-tight version of cycling shorts. They are inbuilt with unique bands that embrace the group of muscles in thighs, glutes and calves. Usually worn under regular shorts, compression shorts protect the pelvis, groin and hips and improve the region's quality of movement.

Calf Guards

Compression calf guards help in compressing the calf muscles along with the foot area. Since these parts of the leg are actively involved in most of the activities, the calf guards can be very helpful in preventing injury and soreness in these regions.

Underwear

Compression underwear is one of the most popular forms of clothing in this category. It provides you with the maximum comfort and security for sensitive body parts, protecting them from pressure and injury. The garment also offers increased support to the concerned regions.

COMPRESSION WEAR—THE TOP 9 BENEFITS

Compression wear has gained immense popularity within the sports community and now in the rehab community, especially in the last few decades. Below I have listed the top reasons this tool is a performance booster.

It improves blood circulation

As I mentioned earlier, compression garments work by exerting gentle pressure on the relevant body parts. Technically, the garment will apply the heaviest pressure on the extremities of the body. The compression, in turn, increases the flow of blood back to the lymph nodes and heart. The phenomenon of better blood circulation has the following beneficial effects on the performance:

- It reduces the overall warm-up time before exercise
- It increases the flow of blood to the muscles, thereby enhancing their ability to contract and stretch

- It prevents the formation of blood clots
- It prevents the occurrence of deep vein thrombosis.

A study conducted as early as 2011 involving young athletes in Australia revealed how wearing compression shorts enhanced blood and oxygen consumption flow amongst runners and triathletes.

It reduces swelling

Compression clothing comes with various advantages for different body parts, especially where swelling and inflammation can happen.

When worn on the upper body, compression wear can apply pressure that can significantly cut down on swelling and inflammation, especially in activities such as weight training.

Compression wear offers vast benefits for the gluteal muscle groups, hips and quadriceps. The gentle pressure exerted by the clothing pushes the blood back to the heart, thereby lowering fatigue considerably.

Calves also benefit from the use of compression stockings, socks and calf guards. It is common for the calf muscles to get swollen after long-standing sessions due to fluid pooling, mainly due to gravity, in the legs. Compression socks can prevent the formation of blood clots and reduce the risk of the development of deep-vein thrombosis.

It reduces the risk of injury

Compression gear regulates the movement of muscles and improves overall flexibility and stability. These factors go a long way in reducing the overall risk of injury to the person, especially during their exercise programs. Specially designing these products to fit the relevant body parts closely provides adequate support and protection, thus helping to avoid injury.

It expedites the rate of recovery

Regular use of compression wear can drastically cut down on the risk of injury and muscle damage.

In related research, Dr John Jakeman of the School of Social and Health Sciences at the University of Abertay Dundee in Scotland reported that using such compression wear impacted the cellular membrane turnover in a damaged muscle group. The use of this compression clothing decreased the inflammatory response to muscle damage, thereby expediting recovery.

It improves the rate of proprioception

Proprioception is typically an individual's perception or sense of how their body positions in space. Our joints have built-in proprioceptors that provide us with information on where our joints are in space. Consistent compression improves this proprioception.

According to experts, a better level of proprioception improves the quality of movement and reduces overall fatigue. It enhances the level of stability.

We've learnt in the above sections about how compression garments work. To expand on this knowledge, when the unique elastic fibre of the fabric envelops muscles in an absolute fit, it lowers the risk of injury considerably. It occurs due to the low vibration and more excellent protection to the relevant forces. Apart from preventing injuries, the increased stability of the muscles will also reduce muscle spasms and pains.

It reduces soreness in muscles

Water retention and swelling are some of the most common reasons for increased muscle soreness and discomfort. Compression clothing provides a higher blood circulation level that helps flush out harmful ingredients such as lactic acid, one of the leading causes of muscle soreness.

According to a study published in the *Journal of Sports Sciences*, compression garments considerably reduced Delayed Onset Muscle Soreness (DOMS). DOMS is common in athletes who feel a muscular ache or soreness up to 48 hours after considerable exercise. DOMS occurs because there is micro-tearing of the muscles used during the given activity or sport. Yet another study amongst cyclists revealed lower levels of lactic acid after wearing compression socks for some time.

It reduces fatigue levels

Good quality compression wear increases the overall rate of blood circulation, therefore delivering more oxygen to the cells. This phenomenon reduces fatigue levels considerably. In addition, tight-hugging clothing also gives a massaging effect to the muscles, which also helps in reducing fatigue levels.

A relevant study amongst runners showed how active people who wore compression socks could run as much as four per cent longer than those who didn't.

It increases the aerobic and anaerobic threshold

Since compression wear can improve the blood flow and oxygen consumption within the body, it can also improve the overall stamina levels. One such study conducted among 21 runners concluded that there was a 2.1–6.2% improvement in the aerobic and anaerobic threshold for those wearing compressions socks.

It offers a psychological boost

There is substantive research to support that using compression wear gives a person a psychological boost. Experts feel that just knowing that they are wearing a protective garment gives them an extra edge of confidence for some people. Having confidence helps improve a person's mindset, and this pushes them towards a positive attitude. And with a positive mindset, the unachievable becomes more achievable.

The Buying Guide

The world of compression can often turn out to be a perplexing one. The last few decades have witnessed a staggering increase in the number of people opting for this type of wear.

In fact, compression wear now accounts for a huge share of the sports apparel market. For this reason, there has been a widespread mushrooming of companies and firms offering various varieties and types of compression wear. However, it is common for people to opt for improper compression clothing, which is either not of the right quality or it does not suit their specific needs for some reason.

In this section you'll find a detailed buying guide, which can help you make the right choice for your compression wear.

THE TOP 5 FACTORS

Make it sport-specific

The most important criteria to bear in mind is your specific activity or sport of choice. It would be best if you had a clear insight into what body parts are involved in your particular activity, including which muscles need maximum protection and so on. Only go in for such compression clothing that will fit your purpose.

Know the manufacturer

It is best to do your own research about the manufacturer in question. Read up as much as you can about the credentials of the manufacturing company involved. Some companies offer vivid details about their manufacturing procedures. Read more about the materials they use and the research that goes behind designing their products. For instance, companies like Supacore back up all their products with years of study and reach medical-grade classification. You will read more about this company in the later sections.

Know your size and fit

It is often a myth that one needs to buy a smaller size of compression wear to fit better. You must remember that the manufacturers have already taken care of this aspect. You must refer to the size chart and only purchase the clothing specifically designed for your body size and measurements.

Know the features

Some brands of compression wear also offer specific advantages such as UV protection and thermal lining. Check out if you want any of these features and whether your chosen product offers these or not.

Know the practicality

Though most compression wear items are made from similar raw materials, you might find some designs difficult to wear, especially in hot weather. Moreover, you also need to ensure that the piece of compressive clothing you are buying will be easy to wear or slip-on, especially in the case of compression socks and stockings.

By now, as a dedicated person to their rehab, you may have been through a fantastic or frustrating journey of finding proper compression wear. Get it right and compression wear may even provide you with a minor miracle for enhancing your rehab or performance. The test to getting the best out of compression wear is to choose your product wisely and do your research before choosing any specific product.

Supacore—The Case Study

This section gives you a detailed insight into one of the world's best manufacturers of compression wear. Having served the medical and sporting community for many years now, Supacore has emerged as one of the most trustworthy brands amongst people. In addition to this, the company also offers unique products in the medical and lifestyle niche. Read on to know more about the brand and why even after so many years, it is still one of the most dependable brands when it comes to compression wear.

Research-based products

At Supacore, the designs of the entire product range follow years of research. The whole structure and composition of the product use medical research and findings. The powers that be at Supacore point out that their products build on the principle of graduated compression, putting the strongest pressure on the areas that require it the most. The research team at Supacore emphasises that when the blood circulates properly, it restores the oxygen and other nutrients back to the tired muscles. For this reason, the Sigvaris compression clothing claims to help the muscles regenerate more efficiently and remove any traces of lactic acid that have built up.

Special features

The product range of Supacore has a few other unique features that make them especially useful and practical. Here, I have listed a few of these features:

- Controlled efficacy compression wear
- Fitted compression to ensure the best product
- Innovations make compression therapy progress, such as CoreTech leggings and shorts, the only patented compression technology that decreases back pain symptoms like osteitis pubis, hamstring, groin, hip and pelvic instability.
- Textile intelligence with a unique sizing system to cover the maximum size range
- A large choice of models, textures and colours to suit varied tastes. It makes the compression as close to custom-fit as you can get for a person.

Recovery—The Hidden Secret

A writer once righteously remarked, 'Recovery is the forgotten component of training'.

Recovery, the term used in the sports jargon, refers to the stage in which the person allows their body to:

- Adapt to the stress of exercise
- Repair damaged muscle and tissue
- Replenish depleted energy reserves

Fundamentally, the Recovery Principle states that every person needs to give adequate time to their body to recuperate after training or competition. In fact, you might consider the stage of recovery to be as important as the exercise or sport itself, as far as boosting performance is concerned.

Experts suggest incorporating at least 36 hours of active recovery between quality sessions. Some of the most effective tools of recovery include:

- Sleep
- Nutrition and Hydration
- Massage
- Physiotherapy
- Low-intensity workouts (such as swimming)
- Stretching
- Posture

You will read more about some of the tools and techniques in the later sections of this book.

The Two Categories

Analysts talk about two different types of recovery stages, including Short-term or active recovery, and Long-term recovery. Read on for a brief explanation of each of these two categories.

(a) Short-term recovery

Short-term recovery is also known as active recovery or immediate recovery. It refers to the recovery period immediately after a spell of intense exercise. This stage occurs immediately after the training or the session of activity is over.

Experts define short-term recovery as the period in which the individual takes up low-intensity exercises to help the body cool down. Active or short-term recovery strongly links to performance benefits. You will read more about this in the later sections of this book.

(b) Long-term recovery

A long-term recovery plan is usually an integral part of a training program. The recovery lasts for days and weeks and is part of the training program to allow for sufficient recovery from injury and stress.

In the long run, both active and long-term recovery plays a crucial role in boosting a person's overall rehab performance.

The Homeostasis Logic

There is a concrete, evidence-based, scientific logic behind the Recovery Principle. Let's take a deeper look into the Recovery Principle before we move on.

The human body is programmed with pre-set levels of certain vital conditions to function normally. In ideal conditions, your body needs to work at a certain pre-set level regarding the following four core aspects:

- Internal body temperature
- Salt conditions
- Nutrient and waste balances
- Acidity

The stage where all the above factors are at the standardised and desirable levels is known as the individuals' level of homeostasis.

After a session of heavy physical exercise, your body gets into the mode of metabolic recovery. It is a stage where your heart will continue to beat at a faster rate, and you will keep on breathing hard for several minutes after your workout or exercise is over. At this stage, your body is undergoing homeostasis in an attempt to return to its pre-set conditions. Failure to return to this stage or maintain homeostasis can result in severe organ malfunction or even failure.

Besides, when you exercise, a series of developments take place within your body. These include the breakdown of muscle tissue, depletion of energy stores or muscle glycogen, and loss of fluid. It is here that recovery time plays a vital role. It helps in replenishing the energy stores and the damaged muscle tissue to repair and rejuvenate.

You will read more about the specific benefits and techniques of recovery in the later sections of the book.

Mind and Soul—The Top 10 Benefits

Recovery offers an enormous range of benefits to you and works in both the short and long term. This section lists out each benefit in detail.

Is vital for maintaining the level of homeostasis

In the above sections, I explained how homeostasis is an essential concept in human body mechanics. A failure to maintain homeostasis can cause serious health issues like organ failure.

It helps the person adapt to higher levels of stress

It is essential to understand the principle of adaption if you want to understand the role of recovery. Every time you increase the intensity of exercise, your body needs to exert as much pressure to cope with it. However, your body will get used to the stress after some time, after which you can further increase the stress level. It is known as the principle of adaption. Alternatively, it is you pushing yourself outside your comfort zone. It is what all those who want to improve performance will do.

Now, the principle of adaption will only come into force if you give your body sufficient time to cope with the additional stress of physical exertion. The recovery period for activity facilitates the accurate implementation of this principle.

It helps the body repair damaged muscle and tissue

It is the essential physiological benefit of the stage of recovery. The human body needs sufficient periods of rest between heavier workouts and activity sessions. It is necessary to allow the body to repair damaged muscles, tendons and ligaments. The recovery time given to the body helps restore the energy-producing enzymes inside the muscle fibres.

This period of low physical activity also helps in the removal of chemicals that might have built up due to the cell activity during physical exercise.

It helps the body replenish energy reserves

When you exercise, your body loses its stores of glycogen. The carbohydrate content stored in the muscles and liver helps you exert during intense physical activity. Both the body's active and long-term recovery periods replenish its energy and fuel reserves with the aid of the right recovery nutrition, foods and fluids.

It encourages protein synthesis

Protein synthesis is an internal body mechanism that helps in:

- Increasing the protein content of muscle cells
- Minimising muscle breakdown
- Increasing muscle size

When consuming the right foods and fluids in the recovery period, protein synthesis is maintained at an optimal level, thereby achieving the above results.

Offers comprehensive psychological benefits

Experts point out the significant psychological benefits of recovery. A poor recovery rate can actually lead to excessive stress, staleness or even burnout in the rehab journey. Your mind and body require sufficient time for rejuvenation and psychological preparation for the forthcoming sessions.

It allows mental preparation

Psychologists consider the recovery period as the most crucial stage of a training program. At this time, the mind can actively concentrate on solving any issues like lack of confidence or excess anxiety. Counsellors and therapists can also actively counsel people recovering from injuries and poor performance in this period. Moreover, this stage is also important to prepare the person for a higher level of activity.

It gives adequate time for retrospection

During these periods of low activity, the person can look back and identify their weaker zones of performance. Once done, they can then work to strengthen these areas for better overall performance in the future.

It prevents venous pooling

Venous pooling is a mechanism in which blood accumulates in the veins of the legs. The arteries in the human body carry blood from the heart to the rest of the body. The veins are responsible for moving the blood back to the heart, while the valves stop the blood from flowing back. Venous pooling will happen when your veins cannot send blood back from the limbs to the heart due to a variety of reasons. Muscle weakness and injury is one reason for venous pooling, which can occur if the body does not have time to recover.

It prevents the development of overtraining syndrome

Due to a lack of guidance, some people see constant training and practice as the only path to success. Hence, they do not give their body enough time to recover from the stress and damage of exercise. In short, they don't listen to their body's symptoms. If this trend continues for too long, it can further lead to a condition known as overtraining, which often results in a cycle of pain and debilitation.

Key Aides to Recovery

As we studied in the above sections, there is a vast range of tools and aides one can use for active and long-term recovery. The means of recovery you choose will depend on the kind of activity you do and its level of intensity. In this section, we discuss some of the essential tools to aid speedy recovery in rehab.

A) Physiotherapy

Back pain, as we know, may be due to injury, biomechanical understanding, mobility, movement patterns and core. Physiotherapy is the most effective tool for recovery, using a careful combination of hands-on techniques, individual assessment, in-depth analysis, and custom-made exercises. Physiotherapy relieves the body of its pains, fatigue and stress.

Also known as physical therapy, this method involves carefully planned and evidence-based patient-specific exercises to solve a wide range of purposes.

Here are a few benefits of physiotherapy as a tool for expediting recovery in back pain:

- It corrects abnormal biomechanics to help improve control, mobility and core
- It helps nerves, muscles and joints to work in synergy
- It helps rebuild strength and endurance in affected muscles
- It helps improve the range of motion, which is vital to the activity
- It enhances the flexibility of joints
- It helps in relaxing tired muscles and joints
- It helps relieve pain and pressure on the joints in the body.

All of the above measures combine to expedite the recovery rate and offer many advantages such as rehabilitation from injury and increased stamina for new events.

B) Massage

Massage is one of the most important tools of recovery. Experts point out that massage evokes a relaxation response, reflected further in a lower resting heart rate (RHR) and balanced blood pressure readings.

The benefits of massage:

- It promotes the blood flow in the body, also leading to better delivery of oxygen and nutrients to muscles, and the removal of toxins
- It leads to better function of the cardiovascular system since the blood vessels get dilated
- It helps the tired muscles to warm up and stretch properly, in turn increasing flexibility and preventing the formation of adhesions and knots
- It improves the flexibility of muscles and joints
- It helps in the breakdown of the scar tissue that might have formed due to previous injuries and trauma
- It helps in overall pain reduction
- It helps reduce fatigue to a great extent
- It offers psychological relaxation
- It eases stiffness in various body parts
- It reduces anxiety and stress that develops in a competitive, everyday environment
- Regular massage during the recovery period will also stimulate your parasympathetic system. It will lead to better dopamine and serotonin levels and reduce the secretion of the cortisol hormone, also known as the stress hormone.

C) Contrast baths

Contrast baths are one of the oldest and most time-tested techniques of recovery in the field of activity. A contrast bath is a technique within the realm of hydrotherapy and immerses the body into cold and warm water alternatively. The method follows the scientific principle of constant and alternate vasodilatation and vasoconstriction. It subjects the body to hot and cold temperatures in turn. It improves blood circulation and helps remove waste materials more effectively away from exercised tissue. For best results, use the following guidelines for contrast baths as a tool for recovery:

- Increase the intensity of the hot and cold water gradually
- Begin with around one minute of heating, then switch. Alternate with one minute hot, one minute cold. Repeat this seven times
- As a general rule, try to keep the hot bath shorter in length than the cold bath
- Try to stretch your muscles more in hot water, but keep moving in the cold to make the cold water more effective
- Always wind up with the cold water
- Decide on what suits you the best. You can either use hot/cold soaks, immersion baths or showers for this method.

Here are some of the most important benefits of a contrast bath, in specific relevance to the stage of recovery in a training program:

- It reduces inflammation and swelling
- It relieves pain related to muscular strains and sprains
- It improves blood circulation
- Research also shows that the body's lactate levels recover faster when using the contrast bath principle.

D) Swimming

Swimming is typically considered the ideal low-intensity workout, best suitable for short-term, active recovery. The activity serves a dual purpose in the context of recovery:

- It relaxes the muscle groups
- It maintains a minimal level of physical activity to keep up the momentum
- Is one of the most desirable cooldown workouts, especially after a session of heavier training.

Here are some of the unique benefits of swimming as a recovery tool:

- Offers relief to the tired joints since water provides soft stimulation
- Is lighter than mild cardio activity and exerts less strain on your muscles and joints
- Repairs the damaged muscle tissue and eases overall stiffness and discomfort
- Increases overall stamina, strength and endurance
- Offers a greater variety than most low-intensity workouts. You can opt for any of the strokes or styles
- Researchers also point out that swimming is an effective recovery method for any person at any activity level.

E) ALTERNATIVE THERAPIES

1. Spinal Manipulation

Spinal manipulation is one of the most widely studied and accepted forms of physiotherapy modalities. Experienced physiotherapists carry out the treatment to alleviate lower back pain. The therapy works based on the assumption that a restricted or maligned spine causes health issues as it hampers the health-maintaining energy flow of the human body.

Experts believe that the human body can heal itself when the spine is aligned and has freedom of movement. Viewing the mind and body as two sides of the equation, this form of treatment pays special attention to the significance of alignment between the spinal cord and the state of health.

How does it work?

There are several techniques used for spinal manipulation. To begin with, to adjust or realign the spine, physiotherapists use hand movements to apply sudden pressure or force on the spine, trying to extend it beyond the normal range of motion. Though such treatments are rarely painful, patients might often hear sounds of cracking or popping sounds in the course of the treatment, which is quite normal and should not be a cause of alarm.

As a secondary technique, the physiotherapists might massage or stretch the muscles to bring about the re-alignment of the spine. Other methods facilitate the spinal re-alignment, including the likes of electrical stimulation, specific exercises, nutrition counselling, and heat and ice therapy.

2. Biofeedback Techniques

In this form of therapy, the practitioner teaches the patient mental and physical exercises while simultaneously monitoring the body using sensors attached to specific points in the body—each of these sensors feeds back to a machine designed to monitor physiological responses.

3. Heat Therapy

Warmth and heat are always associated with comfort and pain relief. However, with lower back pain, heat therapy offers a twin benefit to the patient, i.e. relief from pain and help in healing. Heat therapy is especially beneficial when the cause of lower back pain is a strain and overexertion.

Types of Heat Therapy

1. Dry Heat: In this type of heat therapy, dry heat—such as electric heating pads and saunas—is used to draw out moisture from the body, thus leading to a lot of hydration in the skin.

2. Moist Heat: The typical sources of moist heat are hot baths and humid heating baths, which can considerably facilitate heat's penetration into the muscles.

Common Forms

The most common methods used for heat therapy include hot water bottles, heated gel packs, heat wraps and electric heating pads.

4. Transcutaneous Electrical Nerve Stimulation (TENS)

TENS is a form of complementary therapy that relieves back pain by delivering mild electric pulses to the painful area through the electrodes on the skin. These electrodes stimulate nerve fibres, eventually blocking the pain signals to the brain. Lower back pain mainly responds well to TENS therapy, especially when administered in combination with medical treatments.

F) Alternative Medicine

In problems such as lower back pain, defining a specific cause of the problem may become difficult. In addition, evidence suggests that the conventional forms of medication might not have the desired therapeutic effect on lower back pain. It is in such circumstances that you might want to look at other alternative forms of treatment.

The modalities of alternative therapy generally achieve one or more of the following objectives:

- To relax the tension in muscles
- To rectify the spinal imbalances
- To relieve discomfort
- To ward off risks of long-term problems in the back by improving the strength of the muscles and joint stability.

Read on for a detailed insight into what alternative therapies can help when you are suffering from lower back pain that fails to respond to conventional forms of treatment satisfactorily.

1. Acupuncture

If you are not able to gain satisfactory relief from lower back pain using conventional forms of treatment then acupuncture might offer substantive relief. Medical research shows acupuncture to be an effective form of treatment of lower back pain, having been successfully studied and used over the last few decades.

Acupuncture basically attempts to cure by reducing the level of pain and enhancing the overall state of health. Used as a part of a comprehensive system of healing, known as Oriental Medicine, acupuncture works by stimulation of certain body points along the meridians and channels that are believed to promote blood flow in this stream of alternative therapy.

2. Homeopathy

Homeopathic treatments to obtain relief from lower back pain have been a research subject for quite some time. However, specific homeopathic remedies are most effective in the treatment plan for lower back pain. Read on for a brief listing of each one of these.

- Massage and application of Arnica oil to the sore area
- Oral doses of Arnica or Rhus Toxicodendron
- Bellis perennis for deep muscle injuries.

CHAPTER 5

MEDICAL TREATMENT

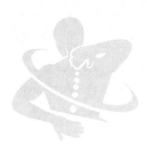

A) CONVENTIONAL MEDICINE

Conventional medicine refers to the cluster of medications most commonly used to obtain relief from human disorders. Traditional forms of medication therapy may be one of the most effective forms of treatments available for lower back pain. However, as with all medications, medicines prescribed for lower back pain also have side effects, which can vary in different cases.

Read on for detailed information on various medication prescribed for lower back pain and their possible side effects, if any, along with any other vital facts the patient needs to know.

1. Painkillers

Painkillers used to obtain relief from LBP are usually divided into two broad categories, including the over-the-counter (OTC) drugs and the more potent medications.

i. Over-the-Counter Medications

Some of the most common OTC medications prescribed for lower back pain include Paracetamolm (Panadol), Ibuprofen (Advil), Naproxen (Naprosyn) and Aspirin.

The above listed OTC drugs are usually safe and do not require a consultation with a medical professional. These are typically considered the first form of medication given for LBP, especially the one lasting for a short time. However, it is not a good idea to use OTC drugs for individuals suffering from the following conditions unless advised otherwise: bleeding, heart problems, kidney disorder and liver problems.

ii. Prescription Drugs

Stronger medications advised for relief from lower back pain include prescription-strength NSAIDs, such as ibuprofen and naproxen. However, opioids are considered the most potent form of pain-relieving medicine and need to be administered under strict medical supervision and only for patients with acute pain. The use of opioids may well result in side effects, including the following: constipation, nausea and sleepiness. In some cases, opioids can also lead to addiction and severe substance abuse.

2. Muscle Relaxants

Muscle relaxants are generally a secondary option to pain-relieving medications and can be helpful, particularly when taken before bedtime, though primarily for shorter durations. Such skeletal muscle relaxants are known to alleviate pain and improve functional ability. However, most of such muscle relaxants come with the possibility of drowsiness and involve care and consideration.

3. Antidepressants

Antidepressants, especially tricyclic antidepressants, are a moderately effective medication for lower back pain. Since depression and anxiety are generally present in patients with lower back pain, this class of drugs can effectively alleviate such symptoms. The most common medications used in this category include Amitriptyline, Nortriptyline, Desipramine, Venlafaxine and Duloxetine. There is evidence that other medications such as Gabapentin and corticosteroids effectively cure lower back pain, though results vary.

The Research

If drugs don't work for back pain, according to studies—what's the answer?

A new study has confirmed the danger of relying too much on drugs to treat back pain. After treating many thousands of people with back pain over the years, at Elite Akademy we aren't surprised. We often see people who are at their wit's end after trying drugs without any improvement.

Rather than rush for drugs, it's always best to locate the underlying cause of back pain by testing what you can and cannot do. The best results come from testing biomechanics, range and quality of movement without any help from drugs.

Most effective long-term treatment involves hands-on physio methods such as correcting biomechanics, exercising, correcting movement, and massage.

The study from Sydney-based The George Institute for Global Health[3] says that 'commonly used non-steroidal anti-inflammatory drugs used to treat back pain provide little benefit, but cause side effects.'

The review has been published in the Annals of the Rheumatic Diseases and reveals only 'one in six patients treated with the pills, also known as NSAIDs, achieve any significant reduction in pain'.

According to the George Institute, earlier research has already demonstrated paracetamol is ineffective, and opioids provide minimal benefit over placebo.

What then is the answer to back pain? Unfortunately, there is no off-the-shelf solution. Everybody is different, and there are many different types and causes of back pain. A professional assessment is the best place to start.

The underlying cause may not be what you expect. It may be posture, it may be an injury, or it may be referred pain from a problem in your body elsewhere. Finding the underlying cause is not possible in a pill packet—it takes time and experience.

Once you know the underlying cause, the solution to easing back pain will vary but will centre around correcting biomechanics, massage, exercise and correct movement.

Back pain sufferers commonly restrict their movements— this is understandable, and it happens subconsciously. To move means pain, so sufferers gradually move less and less without even realising.

Unfortunately, restricting movement is the worst possible thing for your back. We need to move, and this is no more important than with your back.

Recovery needs movement. Once you have found the underlying cause, the next important part of the assessment is

[3]George Institute for Global Health, 2017. *The drugs don't work, say back pain researchers.* [online] ScienceDaily. Available at: www.sciencedaily.com/releases/2017/02/170202090820.html > [Accessed 26 August 2021].

to relieve and prevent pain. It will involve specific stretches and exercises that gradually increase your range of movement.

Many back pain sufferers find that once the pain is under control, they benefit from continuing the exercises and staying mobile. The activity becomes key to preventing further back pain.

So before rushing to use anti-inflammatories like ibuprofen and aspirin next time you have back pain, think about the study and how ineffective these drugs are. Chances are a proper professional assessment will provide more sustained relief and possibly even a life without back pain.

B) SPINAL INJECTIONS

Spinal injections are quite usual as a treatment for lower back pain. Administering injections has two critical objectives in mind, including to alleviate pain and to serve as a diagnostic tool, helping to ascertain the cause of pain.

There are two forms of spinal injections commonly used for relief from lower back pain, including the following:

1. Facet Joint Injections

Facet joint injections aim to decrease inflammation and pain that arises from one or more of the facet joints. Facet joints sit at the back of the spine and are essential for movement and mobility.

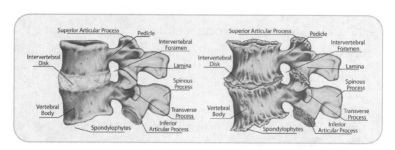

2. Epidural Steroid Injections

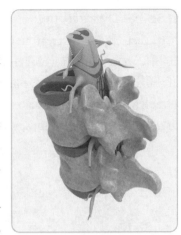

Epidural steroid injections work by injecting pain-relieving medications into the epidural spaces. Once administered, the medicine flows through the epidural space, thereby coating nerve roots and the outer lining of the facet joints.

In addition to the above, other injections are administered into the muscles, soft tissues, and the regions of the deeper back to gain relief from lower back pain. The most common injections amongst these include:

- Trigger point injections, administered by a local anaesthetic into the superficial muscles or soft tissues
- Chemonucleolysis, in which an enzyme is injected into a herniated disc to shrink the disc and relieve pressure on a compressed nerve root
- Prolotherapy, involving an injection of irritant chemicals into soft tissues of the back.

C) SURGICAL INTERVENTION

Surgical procedures are mostly the last option in case of lower back pain. In severe lower back conditions, spinal surgery becomes necessary to relieve the pressure on nerves or alleviate pain in general.

In the following section, we briefly discuss the main types of back surgeries that can relieve lower back pain.

1. Spinal Discectomy

A discectomy is the treatment of herniated discs. The procedure involves removing the soft gel-like material that gets herniated out of the disc, compressing a spinal nerve. Discectomy aims typically at returning the disc to a better and more normal shape. It also tries to relieve the pressure on the spinal nerve located nearby.

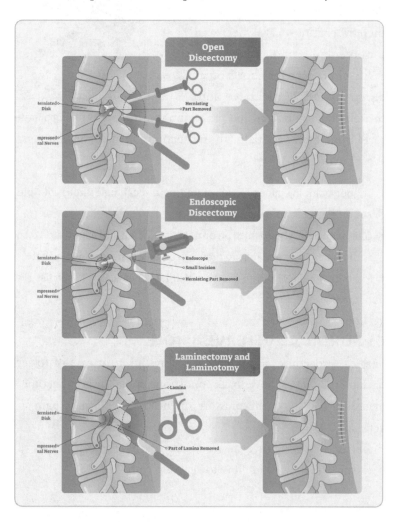

i. Foraminotomy

Foraminotomy is also a back surgery used to relieve the pressure on nerves like discectomy. However, in foraminotomy, the nerve is being pinched for other reasons than merely a herniated disc. Hence, foraminotomy cures the problem by removing a portion of the bone and other related tissue that might compress the nerve.

ii. Laminectomy

This particular procedure relieves the pressure exerted on the spinal cord. Most common conditions that get treated using a laminectomy include spinal stenosis and spondylolisthesis. At times, this particular procedure is done along with spinal fusion to prevent any scope of instability.

2. Spinal Fusion

Spinal fusion is basically surgery linking two or more vertebrae together. A frequent cause of lower back pain is disc space. It is treated effectively with a spine fusion. The surgery aims to remove the movement within the affected portion of the spine, thereby eliminating the primary cause of lower back pain.

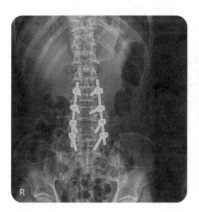 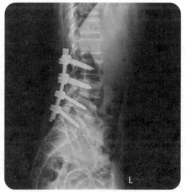

The procedure usually involves instrumentation, including medical devices such as cages, plates, screws and rods, and bone grafts to stabilise the spine. The bone graft materials used generally include:

- Patient's graft (autograft)
- Donor bone (allograft)
- Bone morphogenetic protein (BMP)

3. Spinal Disc Replacement Surgery

Having been recently approved in the USA as an acceptable form of treatment for some types of lower back pain, spinal disc replacement surgery is fast becoming one of the most result-oriented forms of LBP treatments.

The type of surgery involves removing the physical disc or the degenerated disc material. In its place is an implant of an artificial intervertebral disc in the spine. It also helps to know that disc replacement surgery usually is much less invasive than traditional spinal surgery. In fact, the recovery time associated with this type of surgery is generally less than the other forms, such as spine fusion.

Medical Professionals

A series of medical professionals usually need to be involved in a typical treatment plan for lower back pain. Most commonly included medical professionals are:

- Orthopedic surgeons
- Physiotherapists
- Occupational therapists
- Surgical specialists

- Psychologists
- Nurses

Diagnosis

Formulating a result-oriented and effective treatment plan for lower back pain depends mainly on the diagnosis of the condition and the probable cause of the pain.

A scientifically designed diagnostic plan for lower back pain usually comprises of three steps, including:

1 Understanding the patient history
2 Physical examination
3 Imaging procedures

1. Patient History

To begin with, the physician needs to have insight into the patient's medical history. The physician needs to determine any correlation between the current LBP episode and any previous medical history. Various aspects of medical history and information need recording and examining, including:

- Any background or history of heart problems, cancer or arthritis in the family of the patient
- Any history of accidents or injuries that involve the neck, back or hips
- Any signs of conditions like excessive unexplained weight loss or chronic infection
- Any instances where normal activities like coughing, sneezing, exercising or walking aggravate the problem
- Any specific action that might provide respite from the pain, such as lying or sitting down or exercising

- Any previous episodes of back pain
- The pattern of frequency and duration of the pain
- Any specific timing of back pain
- Any problems related to bowel or bladder control
- Any other specific symptoms like morning stiffness, numbness or weakness in the legs.

2. Physical Examination

There is a physical examination of the patient with lower back pain to locate the source of pain and determine the limits of movement caused by it.

In most cases, the patient will perform certain activities and movements that will help diagnose the exact cause and location of the pain.

Main Activities:

- Sit, stand or walk in different ways. The physician observes limitations to activity such as flat-footed, on the toes, on the heels and the like
- Bend forward, backwards and sideways and twisting
- Lift your leg straight up while lying down
- Observe circumference of the calves and thighs that will help in determining any presence of muscle deterioration.

In addition to the above, the physician might also conduct special tests to examine the integrity of nerve functions and reflexes.

3. Imaging Procedures

Conducting a series of imaging procedures helps to point out the exact cause of lower back pain. The precise types of imaging studies carried out depend on the patient's specific signs and the severity of symptoms. If the patient is not suffering from a single underlying cause, then a combination of diagnostic methods might need to be applied.

Here I've listed brief definitions of various kinds of imaging tools used to diagnose lower back pain.

- X-Rays: These are the most common methods that help in detecting the cause and location of back pain and use basic imaging technique
- Magnetic Resonance Imaging (MRI): This process can examine the lumbar region and provide a three-dimensional view of the area. Unlike X-rays, it does not expose the patient to radiation
- Computerised Tomography (CT): A painless procedure used when possible damage to the vertebrae is the cause of lower back pain
- Discography: The process involves injecting a contrast dye into the spinal disc and potentially locating the cause of lower back pain
- Magnetic Resonance Imaging (MRI): A process to examine the lumbar region
- Electrodiagnostic procedures include electromyography (EMG), nerve conductions studies, and evoked potential (EP) studies
- Bone scans: Scans diagnose and monitor infections, disorders in the bone and fractures
- Thermography: This imaging method uses infrared sensing devices to measure minor temperature alterations
- Ultrasound imaging: The procedure uses high-frequency sound waves to obtain images inside the human body.

Prognosis

Research shows the prognosis to be effective in most cases of lower back pain. As many as 80% of the patients recover completely in 4–6 weeks. Meanwhile, the prognosis for patients suffering from chronic pain depends on the actual underlying cause of the pain.

Most often, the effective treatment of lower back pain emanates from a combination of several treatments, in a specific context to the patient's medical history and current symptoms. For instance, one particular patient suffering from LBP might benefit from a combination of massage and medications, while another might get relief from various medication and exercise.

CHAPTER 6

FROM THE YOUNG TO THE ELDERLY

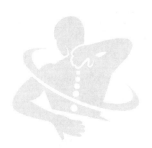

How to prevent back pain in the next generation

Our children are becoming less and less active. It is a shame to see this on such a global scale. The more technologically advanced we become, the more we are losing touch with the games we play as children, and this then results being inactive adolescents and young adults. My clinical work shows that this is a significant contributing factor to lower back pain.

Our bodies need to move. We are dynamic creatures. We must re-teach our kids the importance of playing 2–3 hours per day. Playing sport, running around the yard, riding bikes, dancing, hide and seek—the choices are endless.

When we were growing up, we didn't have the technology to take our focus away. All we had was the games and sports we played outside. For that, I am thankful. But how can we use technology to help our youngsters? We can use it to show them what they are doing. The smartphone is an excellent example. It can take photos, slow-motion video, regular video and time-lapse. What an incredible array of analysis tools our young kids have at their disposal. All the elite athletes I work with get better at what they do because of the analysis they have at their fingertips. They have television replays, video analysis, GoPros. Our kids have these built into their phones! Creating a mindset to analyse sport may help them improve their activity levels, encouraging them to be better, play more and be more active. In turn, it could prevent the severity of sedentary related back problems, which I witness first-hand.

Using current technology is not limited only to helping our children. We can use this technology for our betterment too. We can analyse ourselves—the use of technology to better humankind by improving our form and technique. What an advancement.

Back Pain in Over-60s

Common advice to rest following back pain is needlessly harming over 60s. People are taking longer to get over back pain because of the advice to avoid their sporting activity altogether and rest. But resting is often the worst advice you can get—not only does it slow recovery, but it also prevents you from doing what you love.

Many over 60s are amateur and recreational sportspeople, and there are inevitably instances where back pain will occur. Currently, too many hear that they must cease their sporting activity once injured, out of a misguided view that rest following an injury is the best course.

Our evidence from working with everyone from retirees to Olympians suggests that it's better to stick with your sport at a reduced intensity rather than stay away from that sport altogether.

The current approach to sports injuries is eerily similar to treatment for back pain two decades ago. At that time, physicians recommended bed rest, which turned out to be the worst possible thing to do—patients were miserably inactive and didn't improve.

Now, we know that back pain requires mobility for recovery. Laying on your bed all day just locks the body up and increases the pain. There is a tremendous amount of research, including some good background in the *New England Journal of Medicine*[4].

Inactivity prolongs recovery, which means people are wasting months at a time. There is also a greater risk of regressing.

The best way forward following injury is to slowly ease back into the activity, steadily increasing intensity and duration. You can increase recovery by slowly reintroducing that activity within tolerable comfort levels.

Case Study: Golf Injury

An avid 69-year-old male golfer came to us with a back problem. His previous advice was to give up the game because the walking was too much. After looking at his contributing factors, we found that he could walk four out of the 18 holes. And this is where we started. He would walk every second hole for eight holes and then cart the remaining distance. The approach built up his back conditioning without pushing through pain. Within six months, combined with treatment for his contributing factors, he walked the entire course again.

Case Study: The Walker

I treated a patient who had increased her walking routine dramatically, from almost no walking at all to more than one hour a day quite suddenly. The increase in walking soon resulted in a back injury. The back was painful and made walking almost impossible.

Her initial advice from a GP was to stop walking altogether, yet after two months of inactivity she was still in pain. When the patient attended our clinic, she was at her wit's end.

Mobility was the answer. By gradually increasing walking, combined with physio treatment on the back, the patient could get back her fitness. She learned the hard way that if you don't do any activity, you spiral down rather than building up.

The body needs mobility to recover from any injury, provided it is sensible and part of a program. Rest is usually the worst approach.

[4]Malmivaara, A, et al. 1995. *The Treatment of Acute Low Back Pain — Bed Rest, Exercises, or Ordinary Activity?* | NEJM. [online] New England Journal of Medicine. Available at: <https://www.nejm.org/doi/full/10.1056/NEJM199502093320602> [Accessed 25 August 2021].

CHAPTER 7

THE 'BIG THREE' MISDIAGNOSES HAUNTING BACK PAIN SUFFERERS

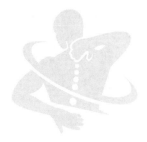

The only thing worse than back pain is prolonging it with incorrect misdiagnosis. Yet this is a common reason why back pain progresses to Chronic Back Pain.

Too many people self-diagnose their pain or, even worse, make an Internet diagnosis. They then become attached to the diagnosis. They often fail to get a second opinion when treatment isn't helping and become resigned to their fate.

It all starts with misdiagnosis, and the 'big three' misdiagnoses that mislead back pain sufferers are:

1. Believing it's a disc problem.

Debilitating disc problems are less common than people think. People are too quick to believe it's a disc. With proper analysis, they often find something completely different, such as gluteal tightness, nerve spasm, lower spine joint tightness or even stress. Around seven out of 10 people, if put under an MRI, would show some disc issue. Our bodies aren't perfect. For example, disc bulges are incredibly common yet don't necessarily cause pain or discomfort. It does not mean the disc is the cause of the back pain.

2. Sciatica

People often assume a shooting nerve-like pain emanating from the back is sciatica—it's a favourite of the self-diagnosed—but nine times out of 10 sciatica is not the issue. Problems can masquerade as sciatica, including lower back biomechanical issues, hip pain and even knee issues. None will improve while you wrongly mistake these complications for sciatica.

3. Stress fractures

Stress fractures can be debilitating and commonly impact sportspeople and those performing physical manual labour. But a funny thing happens to people who suffer from stress fractures— they then fall into the easy routine of blaming any other body issues on the stress fracture, even after it has healed. Meanwhile, they are missing other problems such as shoulder pain, knee problems or neck pain.

Believing that a healed injury is still troubling you is a common trap. It's almost always something else, even if it appears to be mimicking that old familiar pain of a previous injury.

A COMMONLY ASKED QUESTION
Is your back pain coming from your back?
When all is not as it seems.

Nothing seems as easily identifiable as pain, yet it's amazing how often our pain's source hides from us.

We all understand the visceral, uncomfortable, and sometimes unbearable feelings pain brings to us. And when we are in pain, there can be no doubt: if our wrist hurts, we know the pain is in our wrist; if our back hurts, then surely we have a back problem? While pain's experience is immediate and easily located, the pain has other tricks up its sleeve when finding the cause.

It's confusing because when we are in pain's grip, it's hard to accept that pain can be anything other than what it is. But often, the pain we feel is coming from somewhere else in the body. How does this work? It's called 'referred pain', a shared experience increasingly highlighted in much research about pain.

In simple terms, we may consider pain like the engine warning light on your car's dashboard—when something is wrong, the warning light will come on. But we don't necessarily know what the problem is with the motor. If the car needs an examination, we'll take it to a mechanic who will locate the source of the problem.

It's similar to pain because pain often acts as the body's engine warning light—except we will feel the pain somewhere on our body, which is often far from the underlying cause of pain. For example, I treated a patient experiencing debilitating pain in his calf. It was distressing for him because it prevented him from playing soccer with his kids, and the pain became so bad he could barely walk. The patient hobbled into the clinic, where we examined him and found his calf pain had nothing to do with his calf at all. The actual pain source was his back—a classic referred pain example. By treating the back, the patient was soon able to walk freely and play soccer again. No more pain. But if we hadn't identified the underlying back problem, it's easy to see how this pain may have caused long-term issues.

Referred pain is widespread. My physio team find that about 75 per cent of the time, people are experiencing pain beyond where the actual problem lies. If everyone understood their pain is often coming from somewhere else, it would be a significant breakthrough.

People suffering from long-term pain should be encouraged to seek a second opinion. If the original diagnosis is correct, some issues will be chronic and may be challenging to treat. It is also possible that the initial diagnosis is wrong, and you only need to find a trustworthy source of pain for the suffering to ease.

CHAPTER 8

PUTTING IT ALL TOGETHER: 7 TIPS TO MANAGE LOWER BACK PAIN

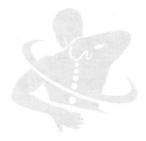

About 80 per cent of us will experience back pain at some point in our lives, with lower back pain the biggest problem. What can we do to manage and prevent this pain?

Most important is remaining as active as possible during lower back pain. It may seem counter-intuitive and may be difficult, but extensive research has confirmed prolonged periods of bed rest worsens lower back pain.

Your body must move. It may be challenging during debilitating bouts of pain—but if you are in pain, the best mantra you can enact is 'little and often'—move a little, as often as you can. Eventually, you can gradually increase your range of movement.

Some other keys to managing lower back pain:

- Watch out for stress: a stressful environment will worsen your back pain. It's natural to worry about how bad your pain is. When it is going to heal and how much it will affect your efficiency, worrying too much will harm you

- Try to practice deep breathing during an attack—feeling tense only makes things worse, so you need to relax your body during periods of pain somehow. Rhythmic and slow breathing works, helping calm your mind as much as possible

- Use a heat or ice pack: heat and ice are most effective when relieving pain. Generally, if an injury is hot to the touch, use ice; if it's cold, use heat. But you may develop a personal preference, so be prepared to try one or the other and stick with it for the first few weeks

- Consider lumbar supports such as back support, corsets and braces— these might also help alleviate pain for some people

- Follow a home exercise program. I cannot stress enough how important it is to keep active and move. Once agreed, the original pain is in place, a home exercise program will help you to progress

- Use pillows. When sleeping, placing a pillow between or under your knees may help your back

- Do light stretching exercises several times a day—it will help with the pain and eventually continue as a preventative measure.

Kusal's quick tips

Even in your everyday life, you can follow some precautions and preventive measures to avoid causing a strain on your back (although I strongly recommend professional advice as well).

Preventive Measures

- Remember not to bend while trying to lift something from the ground. Instead, try to bend your knees and squat to pick up an object. Keeping the back straight, hold the object close to your body and then try to lift it
- While moving heavy objects, try to push instead of pull
- Take frequent breaks to stretch if you need to sit at your desk or drive for longer durations of time
- Follow a regular regimen for exercise as a sedentary and inactive lifestyle contributes to lower back pain substantively

Curative Measures

- Remain as active as possible during lower back pain. Prolonged periods of bed rest have been known to be a causative factor of lower back pain
- Follow a home exercise program soon after the initial pain has subsided.
- Use a heat pad or ice pack (whichever helps you the most) to relieve your pain, especially in the first few weeks
- Lumbar supports such as back support, corsets, and braces might also help alleviate pain
- Try to sleep with a pillow placed between or under your knees

- During an attack of acute back pain, try to practice deep breathing. Rhythmic and slow breathing calms the mind, allowing the body to enter into a more relaxed state
- Try to perform light stretching exercises several times a day
- (A bonus point for over 60s) 'Little and often' is a good mantra— move a little and as often as possible, within tolerable levels of pain. It helps the body recover faster.

Note: Experts strongly warn about creating a stressful environment in context to your lower back pain. Worrying in excess over how bad your pain is, when it is going to heal and how much it will affect your efficiency will harm you all the more instead of offering any healing benefits.

CHAPTER 9

BACK PAIN AND WHY YOU'RE YOUR OWN WORST ENEMY

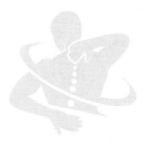

Think you're in tune with your body? Think again. The reality is that most people are their own worst enemies regarding physical well-being. Every week I see people who start with good intentions and unnecessarily hurt themselves by falling for common mistakes. Does this sound like you?

- Going too hard too soon: We live in a 'go hard or go home' culture. But our bodies prefer it if we build fitness and strength gradually.
- Comparing yourself to others: Too many people will start a fitness-related class, which is excellent, and then worry that they aren't as fit/ripped/athletic as the person next to them. They may eventually quit the class, a huge shame. It's important to measure yourself against yourself and not those around you.
- Getting advice and treatment from friends: People's willingness to follow advice from friends who aren't qualified is bewildering. But

every week, people hurt themselves following bogus tips like how to 'crack' your back. Everyone is different—what works for your friend may not work for you. And nobody should 'crack' their back or neck unless they are fond of spinal/stress fractures or plan on an increased risk of stroke.

- Trying to emulate TV and magazines: Celebrity culture is everywhere but has no place in our physical health regime. Unfortunately, people become deluded into chasing an impossible dream. It's pointless trying to emulate celebs—best focus on being the best version of yourself, not someone else.

- Not listening to advice: Think you can cut corners and get away with it? Take an easy example—we learn our whole lives that you must lift heavy objects from the knees, but this doesn't apply to you, right? Why not take a chance on your back?

- Self-diagnosing injuries: Shooting pain in the lower back? It must be sciatica. Can't walk? You've popped a disc. If only actual diagnosis were so simple—but that doesn't stop legions of people performing their diagnosis, or even better, using the Internet or an equally unqualified friend to find the source of their pain. The truth is, getting to the cause of underlying pain can be complex and elusive for trained professionals— so what do you know that they don't?

Finally, remember that making one or more of these mistakes is not a failure—merely a bump on the road to better physical wellbeing. Being aware of these basic mistakes and being honest with yourself will keep you on track. Improve your physical wellbeing and you will be on the road to overcoming your back pain.

Five mental secrets to great exercise

How are your exercise plans going? Are you still persevering or thinking about giving up? Perhaps you've already thrown in the towel? Starting a comprehensive rehab program is hugely rewarding. But it's not easy.

For most people, the mental battle is the real battle. By now, many ambitious exercisers are facing adversity—lack of time, injury, tiredness, you name it. Anyone can face and beat their mental demons provided they know them—even for those who have given up. It's still possible to get going again and salvage something. It's never too late. If you pick it up again and make it through, it will be an achievement, and the results will follow.

If you feel it's a struggle, consider the following five mental secrets commonly used by elite athletes but available to everyone:

- Be flexible: Many exercise regimes falter at the first injury or setback as people struggle to cope with a break in routine. Often people are too ambitious at the outset and need to manage their goals. Flexibility will allow you to adapt and keep going. You will encounter roadblocks, you may need to change routine, but if you stay positive and see it as part of the journey, you'll be better able to accommodate these changes.

- Embrace effort: There are times when the struggle seems overwhelming, mainly if you have set yourself big goals. For example, you may be preparing long-term for a big event. Breaking it down into smaller, achievable lots can provide a big psychological boost. Progress may not always be as fast as you like, but by always remembering where you came from, you'll appreciate the effort and be optimistic about keeping it up.

- Welcome criticism: You may encounter some criticism, perhaps from trainers, team-mates or exercise partners, but provided it's constructive and from someone you trust then a positive mindset will enable you to take it on board, learn from it and improve. It is something elite athletes do exceptionally well.

- Enjoy others' success: Ego can be very destructive in fitness. Especially as you struggle through pain, a healthy mindset will always work wonders. Learn to appreciate and admire your peers' achievements and understand that it is no reflection on us. In fact, we can use it for inspiration.

- Find like-minded partners: Having a workout buddy can be a huge help, but you must be working out with someone on the same page as you who shares a positive mindset and can help push you to new heights. Avoid adopting workout buddies who are negative or drag you down.

How can exercise help reduce chronic pain?

In Australia, one in five people experiences chronic pain. Pain becomes chronic if it takes longer than the expected time to heal. It's important to understand that 'chronic' means longer duration and not the severity of the quality of the pain. Many people unused to this concept are surprised when the pain levels continue, although the injury has healed.

Why does chronic pain occur?

Pain in our bodies is a reliable protective mechanism to prevent us from doing further damage. Pain doesn't just involve the area of injury, but it includes the whole nervous system—your brain, nerves and neural pathways.

If I use an example like lower back pain, the brain's warning signal says that you have not correctly used your body.

You'll undoubtedly get treatment on the back to correct the tissue damage, improve strength and correct the biomechanics.

The brain, however, remembers that a particular incident caused the pain. So every time you're even close to conducting that activity, the brain goes into protective mode and creates the pain as the warning signal.

The tissues usually heal in about six weeks, but this is a yo-yo effect, with the pain continuing until the brain decides that there's no danger. Unfortunately, this process can take time and can minimise your window of movement and activity terribly.

So how can exercise help?

In my experience, the mantra to use is: any movement is an improvement. Do as little as possible without exacerbating that pain signal. And over time, the pain settles as the brain learns that there's no danger.

Try and create movement in different environments. For example, you may not exercise in a gym because the pain levels start quickly and don't subside. However, you could use hydrotherapy as an option because it's gentle on the body.

I'd also recommend starting a diary to plan your weeks according to treatment, recovery, relaxation and wellbeing. For example, head to the physio on Monday, mark in hydrotherapy for Tuesdays and Friday and so on. And as you progress, adjust activity levels to help overcome the pain.

It's important to note that you can overcome chronic pain with a multidisciplinary approach: physio, GP, personal trainer, dietitian, psychologist.

CHAPTER 10

THE K-THEOREM

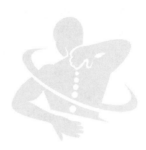

To recap on the preceding chapters, the 'K-Theorem' consolidates this information for you. K-Theorem is composed of four pillars:

Pillar 1. The Performance Pyramid

The body is composed of nerves, muscles, joints and ligaments. These constituents need to function correctly (for the pyramid 'Biomechanics' base to be solid). It then improves flexibility, which then allows for better movement control (quality of movement). Once we have these components, then we need to build upon a good core. And once we have the biomechanical constituents in order, flexibility, quality of movement, and a functioning core, we need to continue building upon strength and conditioning.

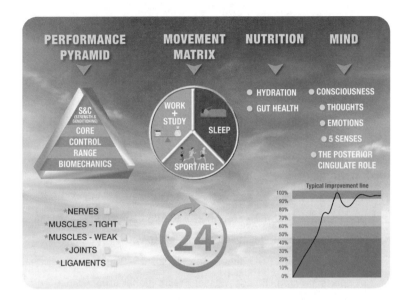

Pillar 2. The Movement Matrix

Once we have a fantastic Performance Pyramid, it has to go to 'work' in a 24-hour cycle. The cycle is composed of Sleep, Work and Recreation/Sport.

Sleep

- The quality and quantity of sleep is essential
- Look out for the age of your mattress and your pillow height.

Work

- Posture, Posture, Posture! It is vital to understand that (poor) posture plays a significant role in pain levels and the onset of your back pain
- The dangers of passive/slouched postures and its effects on our hormones. Good posture increases feel-good hormones. Poor posture increases stress hormones

- Ergonomics matters to people who work at a desk, in a factory, or at home. Get this right, and your body and mind will thank you.

Recreation and Sport

- Doing activities that you love is critical. If you don't love it, you are less likely to follow through with it. The more likely you follow through with it, the better it is for your system.

Mixing things up is essential

- Low-intensity exercises (4–6 days a week), e.g. walking around the block. Perceived intensity around 2–3/10. When doing these activities, you should be able to talk to a person next to you
- Moderate Intensity (2–3 times per week), 45–90-minute sessions, e.g. sports training, fitness classes, recreational sport with friends. Perceived intensity around 5–7/10. Talking to a person next to you is a little more challenging
- High Intensity (2 times per week) around 12 minutes per week! High-Intensity Interval Training. Perceived intensity around 8–9.5/10
- Intensities are so high that you cannot carry a conversation with someone.

Once again, when you mix it up, it helps the rehab process.

Pillar 3. Nutrition

Understand the latest nutrition—plant-based diets and gut health is where the current research is heading. The importance of having a balanced diet is vital. Remember, fads can be dangerous and counterproductive for your rehab goals. These are short-lived and won't help you.

Some old school thinking

10,000 steps used to be a benchmark. It has been one of the best marketing tools to date. It came out of Japan, and there was no research behind it. What we know clinically is that it's far better to mix and match Low, Medium and High-Intensity activities rather than doing 10,000 steps every day. Research shows that even up to 4,000 steps is excellent as long as you mix in some medium and high-intensity exercise. Why is this so? Pushing the body and the human mind outside its comfort zone allows it to grow. We are not static beings—we need to push ourselves to achieve our best results. Follow the Light, Moderate and High-Intensity routines mentioned above for better and lasting results.

Pillar 4. The Human Mind

You must have an understanding of how pain works in the body. The latest knowledge of chronic pain and managing it paves the way for you to overcome it. Remember, stress plays a big part in pain. The connection between high levels of stress and how it transmutes to physical pain is getting a better understanding in the Western world.

The Rock Band and the Tsunami

Putting it all together:

1. The Performance Pyramid is like band members ready to play music.

2. The Movement Matrix is then the band playing beautiful music.

3. When you get nutrition right, it's like the band playing beautiful music in a perfect arena. It is a lovely experience for all!

4. The mind, however, is like a tsunami. A tsunami can wipe out the venue, the music and the musicians. So what goes on in the grey matter is critical!

But the body and mind work hand in hand. You can push the body to improve the grey stuff—enhancing the mind can move the body. Understanding that both these factors are connected is the most important factor in helping your body heal.

Well, all in all, that's the crux of solving back pain. My work over the decades has allowed me to understand the body and mind, and I hope I have been able to bring you some of this insight to help you. I wish you well. Take care and my best to you.

THE LAST WORD

Patient participation is crucial to the success of a treatment program for lower back pain. Intimidating as it might sound, lower back pain is undoubtedly within the realms of treatment and cure, especially if detected early. The right decisions taken in time and reported to the right medical professionals can save you a lifetime of pain and misery, not to mention the loss of efficiency you might have to face due to your nagging pain.

Get set and educate yourself about your symptoms, causes and the treatment choices available to you. The cure and relief are for you to pursue. Science has surely left no stone unturned to devise result-oriented treatment modalities, and it's time you, as a learned individual, begin to seek maximum benefits from such blissful gifts of modern life.

BACK PAIN JOURNAL

	QUESTIONS TO ASK YOURSELF	TICK THE APPROPRIATE CHOICE		
1	On which side do you feel the LBP most often?	Left	Right	
2	How do you classify your LBP?	Dull	Sharp	
3	Have you suffered from LBP before?	Yes	No	
4	How did the LBP start?	Suddenly	Gradually	
5	Have you suffered from any of these?	Injury	Accident	
6	Were you doing any of these activities before LBP started?	Lifting/ Bending	Working on the computer	Driving for long hours
7	Is your current LBP different from any previous episode of LBP you've had?	Yes	No	No LBP earlier
8	Are you aware of the causes of the previous episodes of LBP?	Yes	No	No LBP earlier
9	How long is each episode of LBP?	30 minutes –1 hour	1–5 hours	More than 5 hours
10	Apart from LBP, do you feel pain in any of these parts?	Hip/Thigh	Leg/Feet	
11	Apart from LBP, do you have any of the following?	Numbness/ Tingling	Loss of function in any other part of the body?	Weakness
12	Do long periods of any of these activities aggravate your LBP?	Lifting/ Twisting	Standing/Sitting	Any other
13	Which therapy makes you feel better?	Medicines	Exercise	
14	Are you experiencing any of these symptoms?	Weight loss	Fever	Change in urination/ bowel habits

ABOUT THE AUTHOR

Kusal Goonewardena has established a successful career in building three innovative sports medicine clinics in Melbourne, Australia. His passion is to provide the best solutions in the sports physiotherapy healthcare sector so that patients, athletes and clients continuously receive the most important aspect in health: Results. His passion is to lead practitioners so they live a life of service that is judged by expertise, results, service and education.

Kusal believes that every sports medicine practitioner is in a position to change the lives of athletes and regular people by having the mindset to achieve results in three sessions or less. Kusal states that striving to be their best, living in the moment and continuous perfection of skill acquisition are the keys to his team's success.

Kusal is a 'hands on' leader, combining his business acumen with his outstanding skills as a sports physiotherapist, and he loves leading from the front. With over 65,000 treatments in sports physiotherapy over two decades, he has mentored over 1,000 therapists from around the world. Currently the head of Sports Medicine at Elite Akademy Sports Medicine at the University of Melbourne, he and his team have helped the university achieve a top 5 finish at the prestigious Australian University Games since 2008. His services are on full display when his athletes perform at the Olympics and Winter Olympics for their respective countries.

He is a renowned speaker and has presented in Australia, Singapore, China, Japan and Sri Lanka.

Follow Kusal and Elite Akademy Sports Medicine online

www.eliteakademy.com/

 EliteAkademy

 elite_akademy